The Role of Bioactive Compounds in Human Health and Diseases (2nd Edition)

The Role of Bioactive Compounds in Human Health and Diseases (2nd Edition)

Guest Editor

Jacqueline Isaura Alvarez-Leite

MDPI

Basel • Beijing • Wuhan • Barcelona • Belgrade • Novi Sad • Cluj • Manchester

Guest Editor
Jacqueline Isaura
Alvarez-Leite
Departamento de Bioquímica
e Imunologia
Universidade Federal de
Minas Gerais
Belo Horizonte
Brazil

Editorial Office
MDPI AG
Grosspeteranlage 5
4052 Basel, Switzerland

This is a reprint of the Special Issue, published open access by the journal *Nutrients* (ISSN 2072-6643), freely accessible at: https://www.mdpi.com/journal/nutrients/special_issues/D3N8K855R2.

For citation purposes, cite each article independently as indicated on the article page online and as indicated below:

Lastname, A.A.; Lastname, B.B. Article Title. *Journal Name* **Year**, *Volume Number*, Page Range.

ISBN 978-3-7258-5367-0 (Hbk)
ISBN 978-3-7258-5368-7 (PDF)
https://doi.org/10.3390/books978-3-7258-5368-7

Contents

About the Editor

Jacqueline Isaura Alvarez-Leite

Jacqueline Isaura Alvarez-Leite is a physician specialized in Nutritional Medicine, with a Ph.D. in Biochemistry and Immunology from the Federal University of Minas Gerais (UFMG). She completed her doctoral internship at INRA-France and technical internship at NIH-USA, along with postdoctoral research at Harvard Medical School. She is a Full Professor at UFMG, leading the Laboratory of Atherosclerosis and Nutritional Biochemistry (LABIN-UFMG) and coordinating the Nutritional and Nutritional Therapy Team for Extreme Obesity (ETNNO/UFMG). Her research focuses on Nutritional Biochemistry, particularly antioxidants, obesity, atherosclerosis, and inflammatory bowel diseases.

Preface

We present the reprint "Bioactive Compounds in Health and Disease". Designed for researchers and healthcare professionals, this reprint emphasizes the antioxidant, anti-inflammatory, and antimicrobial properties of bioactive compounds found in foods and herbs. Our goal is to provide valuable and innovative insights into their mechanisms of action and therapeutic potential in health and disease.

Jacqueline Isaura Alvarez-Leite
Guest Editor

nutrients

MDPI

Editorial

The Role of Bioactive Compounds in Human Health and Diseases (2nd Edition)

Jacqueline I. Alvarez-Leite

Departamento de Bioquímica e Imunologia, Universidade Federal de Minas Gerais, Avenida Antônio Carlos 6627, Belo Horizonte 31270-901, Minas Gerais, Brazil; alvarez@ufmg.br

The increasing recognition of bioactive compounds as influential agents in human health has ushered in a new era in nutrition science. These naturally occurring molecules—present in a wide variety of plant- and animal-based foods—are now at the forefront of the discussions surrounding preventative nutrition, functional foods, and integrative therapeutic strategies. Mounting evidence highlights their capacity to modulate critical biological processes, offering potential benefits in mitigating the progression of chronic non-communicable diseases (NCDs), such as obesity, type 2 diabetes, cardiovascular diseases, intestinal diseases, cancer, and neurologic conditions [1,2]. This Special Issue of Nutrients brings together original research and reviews that delve into the uses of bioactive compounds across diverse pathological settings. The works featured herein reflect the interdisciplinary momentum surrounding this field, bridging molecular nutrition, pharmacology, immunology, and clinical practice.

Shimizu et al. (contribution 1) conducted a randomized, double-blind, placebo-controlled clinical trial titled "Preliminary Data on the Senolytic Effects of Agrimonia pilosa Ledeb. Extract Containing Agrimols for Immunosenescence in Middle-Aged Humans". Agrimonia pilosa Ledeb., or Pilosa Cocklebur, is a plant of the family Rosaceae used in Chinese medicine that contains bioactive compounds, such as phloroglucinols, flavonoids, tannins, and phenols, among others. The study assessed whether an extract standardized in agrimols (APE) could reduce senescent $CD8^+$ T cells in adults aged 40–59. While the primary outcomes were not statistically significant across the full cohort after eight weeks of supplementation, exploratory analysis revealed promising immunomodulatory effects in male participants, specifically, reductions in senescent $CD8^+$ cells, increases in naïve T cells, and declines in effector memory populations. These findings, though preliminary, underscore the therapeutic potential of APE as a nutritional senolytic agent and reinforce the importance of bioactive compounds in mitigating age-related immune dysfunction.

Ma et al. (contribution 2) contributed a compelling in vitro study investigating metabolic regulation in a HepG2 steatosis model mimicking metabolic dysfunction-associated steatotic liver disease (MASLD). By tracing carbon flux using ^13C-labeled glucose, the authors evaluated the effects of several flavonoids—naringenin, morin, silibinin, and topiramate—on key metabolic pathways. Silibinin and topiramate significantly reduced lipid accumulation and suppressed de novo palmitate synthesis, potentially via the modulation of the pyruvate dehydrogenase (PDH) pathway. In contrast, morin enhanced lipogenesis and inhibited ribose synthesis. The oleic acid-induced model demonstrated that glucose utilization favored lipid storage at the expense of ribose production and fatty acid desaturation. Given that the compound concentrations were aligned with human exposure levels, these metabolic modulations may reflect physiologically relevant outcomes. Nonetheless, future preclinical and clinical research is warranted to explore therapeutic

 https://doi.org/10.3390/nu17142279

windows, treatment duration, and stage-specific efficacy across MASLD and its progression to MASH.

This Special Issue also welcomes innovative contributions that bridge traditional herbal wisdom with contemporary pharmacological insight. In the study by Budriesi et al. (contribution 3), the authors present HEMEO, a composite formulation composed of herbal extracts (*Asparagus racemosus, Tabebuia avellanedae*, and *Glycyrrhiza glabra*) and essential oils (*Foeniculum vulgare, Mentha piperita*, and *Pimpinella anisum*), each rich in bioactive constituents like saponins, flavonoids, glycyrrhizin, menthol, and anethole. Ex vivo analysis using isolated guinea pig tissues revealed that HEMEO selectively modulates ileal and colonic motility, with potential relevance to functional gastrointestinal disorders. Moreover, HEMEO showed antibacterial activity against *Helicobacter pylori*, and antioxidant potential, suggesting its multifaceted role as a gastrointestinal health supplement. While the individual ingredients are pharmacologically well characterized, their synergistic combination opens up new avenues for translational research—particularly in the management of motility disturbances, inflammation, and microbial imbalance.

In a complementary direction, Ávila et al. (contribution 4) explored the cardiometabolic benefits of capsaicin, a pungent alkaloid derived from chili peppers. Utilizing an ApoE-deficient mouse model, the authors demonstrated that capsaicin supplementation attenuates atherosclerotic lesions, improves lipid profiles, and reduces systemic inflammation. Mechanistic insights revealed the modulation of cholesterol transport, marked by decreased foam cell formation through the downregulation of scavenger receptor A and upregulation of ABCA1-mediated efflux. These effects were largely dependent on TRPV1 receptor activation, with a complex interaction involving PPARγ. The study offers preclinical support for capsaicin's anti-atherogenic potential and illustrates the broader theme of dietary compounds acting on nuclear and membrane-bound signaling pathways to influence chronic disease outcomes.

To further enrich this editorial, Lee et al. (contribution 5) published their study, which explores the immunomodulatory capacity of *Euglena gracilis*, a unicellular alga rich in β-1,3-glucan paramylon. Using an in vitro model and a cyclophosphamide-induced immunosuppressed mouse model, supplementation with *E. gracilis* powder restored innate and adaptive immune markers, reversing weight loss, normalizing splenic lymphocyte profiles, and increasing pro-inflammatory cytokines and serum IgM levels. Notably, the hepatic expression of dectin-1—a key receptor in β-glucan-mediated immune activation—was upregulated. These findings highlight *E. gracilis* as a promising natural immunostimulant, particularly under immunocompromised conditions.

Yimam et al. (contribution 6) further addressed immune restoration using UP446, a standardized bioflavonoid composition derived from *Scutellaria baicalensis* and *Acacia catechu*. In mouse models of oxidative stress-accelerated immunosenescence and chemically induced immune suppression, the oral administration of UP446 enhanced NK and T cell responses, antioxidant capacity, and thymic integrity, while suppressing NFκB and restoring IgA and IgG levels. These findings support the potential of UP446 in preserving respiratory and systemic immune resilience, particularly in aging or environmentally stressed populations.

Also featured is the study by Shin et al. (contribution 7), which evaluated the antihypertensive effects of *Lindera erythrocarpa*, leaf ethanolic extract (LEL). Vascular reactivity and in vivo blood pressure assessments revealed that LEL exerts vasodilatory action via the activation of NO–cGMP signaling, calcium channel blockade, and potassium channel opening, coupled with angiotensin II inhibition. Oral dosing reduced systolic and diastolic pressures in hypertensive rats, pointing to LEL's potential as a multi-target natural therapy for hypertension, pending further safety and mechanistic studies.

Finally, Gonda et al. (contribution 8) addressed an emerging post-pandemic concern: diabetes onset in elderly individuals following COVID-19 infection. In patients aged 80 years and older, those who received *Ficus pumila* L. extract—a traditional Okinawan remedy—showed improved HOMA-β and HOMA-IR indices, indicating an enhanced insulin secretory function and reduced resistance. This study opens up new avenues for the use of plant-based interventions in supporting glycemic control in vulnerable, post-COVID populations.

Altogether, this Special Issue of Nutrients presents a multidimensional exploration of how bioactive compounds interact with key physiological systems, from immunity and metabolism to vascular and endocrine health. The breadth of therapeutic targets and mechanistic insights represented here underscores the role of dietary bioactives as more than just supportive agents; they are foundational tools in the design of personalized, preventative, and integrative health strategies.

Conflicts of Interest: The authors declare no conflict of interest.

List of Contributions:

1. Shimizu, Y.; Shimodan, S.; Hayashida, M.; Yazaki, M.; Sakurada, T.; Watanabe, T.; Ishii, Y.; Hirose, Y.; Saito, J.; Teramoto, S. Preliminary Data on the Senolytic Effects of *Agrimonia pilosa* Ledeb. Extract Containing Agrimols for Immunosenescence in Middle-Aged Humans: A Randomized, Double-Blind, Placebo-Controlled, Parallel-Group Comparison Study. *Nutrients* **2025**, *17*, 667. https://doi.org/10.3390/nu17040667.
2. Ma, L.; Lu, Q.-Y.; Lim, S.; Han, G.; Boros, L.G.; Desai, M.; Yee, J.K. The Effect of Flavonoids and Topiramate on Glucose Carbon Metabolism in a HepG2 Steatosis Cell Culture Model: A Stable Isotope Study. *Nutrients* **2025**, *17*, 564. https://doi.org/10.3390/nu17030564.
3. Budriesi, R.; Corazza, I.; Roncioni, S.; Scanferlato, R.; De Luca, D.; Marzetti, C.; Gotti, R.; Rizzardi, N.; Bergamini, C.; Micucci, M.; et al. Herbal Extracts Mixed with Essential Oils: A Network Approach for Gastric and Intestinal Motility Disorders. *Nutrients* **2024**, *16*, 4357. https://doi.org/10.3390/nu16244357.
4. Ávila, D.L.; Fernandes-Braga, W.; Silva, J.L.; Santos, E.A.; Campos, G.; Leocádio, P.C.L.; Capettini, L.S.A.; Aguilar, E.C.; Alvarez-Leite, J.I. Capsaicin Improves Systemic Inflammation, Atherosclerosis, and Macrophage-Derived Foam Cells by Stimulating PPAR Gamma and TRPV1 Receptors. *Nutrients* **2024**, *16*, 3167. https://doi.org/10.3390/nu16183167.
5. Lee, H.H.; Seong, J.-Y.; Kang, H.; Cho, H. *Euglena gracilis* Enhances Innate and Adaptive Immunity through Specific Expression of Dectin-1 in CP-Induced Immunosuppressed Mice. *Nutrients* **2024**, *16*, 3158. https://doi.org/10.3390/nu16183158.
6. Yimam, M.; Horm, T.; O'Neal, A.; Chua, P.; Jiao, P.; Hong, M.; Jia, Q. Botanical Bioflavonoid Composition from *Scutellaria baicalensis*- and *Acacia catechu*-Protected Mice against D-Galactose-Induced Immunosenescence, and Cyclophosphamide Induced Immune Suppression. *Nutrients* **2024**, *16*, 3144. https://doi.org/10.3390/nu16183144.
7. Shin, S.; Park, J.; Choi, H.-Y.; Bu, Y.; Lee, K. Antihypertensive Effects of *Lindera erythrocarpa* Makino via NO/cGMP Pathway and Ca^{2+} and K^{+} Channels. *Nutrients* **2024**, *16*, 3003. https://doi.org/10.3390/nu16173003.
8. Gonda, K.; Hai, T.; Suzuki, K.; Ozaki, A.; Shibusa, T.; Takenoshita, S.; Maejima, Y.; Shimomura, K. Effect of *Ficus pumila* L. on Improving Insulin Secretory Capacity and Resistance in Elderly Patients Aged 80 Years Old or Older Who Develop Diabetes After COVID-19 Infection. *Nutrients* **2025**, *17*, 290. https://doi.org/10.3390/nu17020290.

References

1. Kussmann, M.; Cunha, D.H.A.; Berciano, S. Bioactive compounds for human and planetary health. *Front. Nutr.* **2023**, *10*, 1193848. [CrossRef] [PubMed]
2. Kurek, M.; Benaida-Debbache, N.; Elez Garofulić, I.; Galić, K.; Avallone, S.; Voilley, A.; Waché, Y. Antioxidants and Bioactive Compounds in Food: Critical Review of Issues and Prospects. *Antioxidants* **2022**, *11*, 742. [CrossRef]

nutrients

MDPI

Brief Report

Effect of *Ficus pumila* L. on Improving Insulin Secretory Capacity and Resistance in Elderly Patients Aged 80 Years Old or Older Who Develop Diabetes After COVID-19 Infection

Kenji Gonda [1,2,3,*], Takeshi Hai [4], Kouichi Suzuki [3,4], Akihiko Ozaki [1,2], Takashi Shibusa [5], Seiichi Takenoshita [6], Yuko Maejima [3] and Kenjyu Shimomura [3]

1 Department of Breast and Thyroid Surgery, Jyoban Hospital of Tokiwa Foundation, Iwaki City 972-8322, Fukushima, Japan; ozakiakihiko@gmail.com
2 Department of Gastrointestinal Tract Surgery, Fukushima Medical University, 1 Hikarigaoka, Fukushima City 960-1295, Fukushima, Japan
3 Department of Bioregulation and Pharmacological Medicine, Fukushima Medical University, 1 Hikarigaoka, Fukushima City 960-1295, Fukushima, Japan; suzukou8931@gmail.com (K.S.); maejimay@fmu.ac.jp (Y.M.); shimomur@fmu.ac.jp (K.S.)
4 Department of Internal Medicine, Daido Central Hospital, 1-1-37 Asato, Naha City 902-0067, Okinawa, Japan; 81takeshi@gmail.com
5 Department of Internal Medicine, Jyoban Hospital of Tokiwa Foundation, Iwaki City 972-8322, Fukushima, Japan; takashi-shibusa@tokiwa.or.jp
6 Department of Drug Research for Astatine-221 Targeted Alfa Therapy, Fukushima Medical University, 1 Hikarigaoka, Fukushima City 960-1295, Fukushima, Japan; akiko-t@fmu.ac.jp
* Correspondence: gondake@fmu.ac.jp; Tel.: +81-246-81-5522

Abstract: (1) Background: It has been reported that people affected by COVID-19, an infectious disease caused by SARS-CoV-2, suffer from various diseases, after infection. One of the most serious problems is the increased risk of developing diabetes after COVID-19 infection. However, a treatment for post-COVID-19 infection diabetes has not yet been established. In this study, we investigated the effects of *Ficus pumila* L. extract, which has traditionally been used to reduce blood glucose levels in Okinawa, on patients who developed diabetes after COVID-19 infection. (2) Methods: In total, 128 rehabilitation patients aged 80 years old or older who developed diabetes after COVID-19 infection were included. The HOMA-β (Homeostatic model assessment of β-cell function) and HOMA-IR (Homeostatic model assessment of insulin resistance) were assessed to evaluate the glucose tolerance. (3) Results: The HOMA-β decreased and HOMA-IR increased in patients who developed after diabetes after COVID-19 infection. Subsequently, 59 patients were given *Ficus pumila* L. extract and their HOMA-β and HOMA-IR improved after ingestion. On the other hand, the control group of patients who did not consume *Ficus pumila* L. showed no improvement in both HOMA-β and HOMA-IR. (4) Conclusions: *Ficus pumila* L. extract, ingested by patients who developed diabetes after COVID-19 infection, stimulated insulin secretion capacity and improved insulin resistance.

Keywords: *Ficus pumila* L.; diabetes mellitus; COVID-19; HOMA-β; HOMA-IR

1. Introduction

A large study based on approximately 200,000 people found that patients infected with COVID-19 by SARS-CoV-2 have an increased risk of developing diabetes within a year, unrelated to the severity of symptoms upon infection [1,2].

It has been reported that patients with no previous risk factors for diabetes are also more likely to develop diabetes after infection. Patients who develop diabetes after infection resemble those with type 2 diabetes mellitus, and have been reported to have both impaired insulin secretion and increased insulin resistance, which are two major causes of type 2 diabetes mellitus.

Ficus pumila L. is native to East Asia (China, Japan, and Vietnam) and belongs to the mulberry family in Figure 1a,b. *Ficus pumila* L. was named by the botanist Carl von Linne. In Japan, *Ficus pumila* L. is found only in Okinawa, where an internationally recognized area has outstanding longevity. The extracts of *Ficus pumila* L. have been traditionally consumed in Okinawa for more than 500 years to promote their health [3] in Figure 1c,d. In Okinawa, people drank tea made from the extraction of *Ficus pumila* L. plants for their health for more than 500 years. Now, this kind of tea is extremely rare.

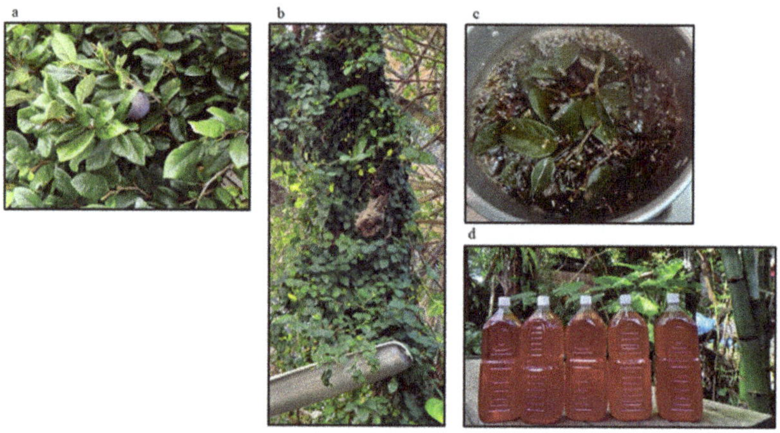

Figure 1. Close-up of the leaves, the extracts of Ficus pumila. (**a**) Leaves, stems, and fruits of *Ficus pumila* L. (**b**) *Ficus pumila* L. commonly known as the creeping fig or climbing fig around trees in nature is a species of flowering plant in the mulberry family. (**c**) Boiling washed leaves and stems of *Ficus pumila* L. in Motobu water. (**d**) *Ficus pumila* L. in the Motobu area of Okinawa Prefecture was carefully made into amber-colored Ficus pumila tea.

In our study, *Ficus pumila* L. showed therapeutic efficacy in hypertension, hyperlipidemia, and hyperuricemia [3]. The reason for the use of *Ficus pumila* L. extract in the treatment of patients who developed diabetes after COVID-19 infection was that it was inferred that *Ficus pumila* L. has antiviral and antidiabetic effects [4,5]. We have not conducted enough research on normal people or people with diabetes who do not have COVID-19 and who are taking *Ficus pumila* L. extract. This is because if patients are taking antiglycemic medication or using insulin, there is a risk of hypoglycemia symptoms if patients ingest Ficus pumila L. extract. In this study, the history of oral use and insulin use are strictly excluded.

The bioactive compounds of *Ficus pumila* L. and the latest knowledge on treatments were reported in detail. Polyphenols (Rutin, Apigenin, Luteolin, Quercetin, Kaempferol), have so far been extracted from *Ficus pumila* L. leaves, stems, and fruits, and these bioactive compounds exhibit multiple therapeutic activities [6] in Figure 2a–e. However, it is now consumed only in certain areas of the main island, and its existence is unknown even to the islanders.

In the present study, we examined whether extracts from *Ficus pumila* L. are effective in improving the hyperglycemia of diabetic patients after COVID-19 infection.

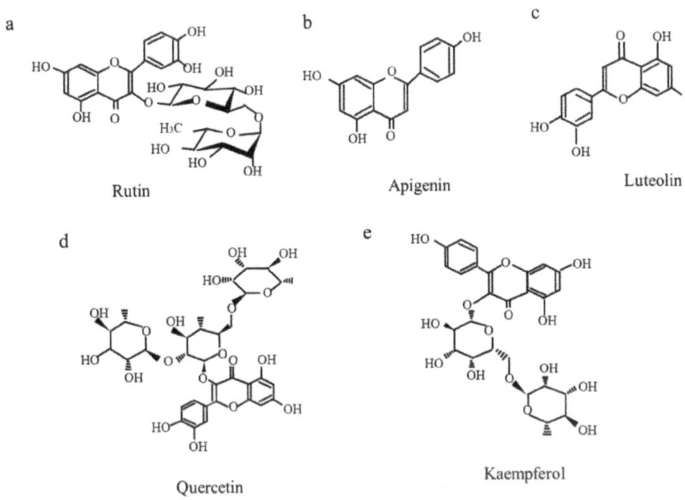

Figure 2. Bioactive polyphenol compounds. (**a**) Rutin, (**b**) Apigenin, (**c**) Luteolin, (**d**) Quercetin, and (**e**) Kaempferol have been extracted from *Ficus pumila* L. leaves and stems.

2. Materials and Methods

2.1. Preparation of the Extract

The source of the *Ficus pumila* L. plant was the Motobu region of Okinawa Prefecture. *Ficus pumila* L. grows in the Motobu region of Okinawa Prefecture. Okinawa is a subtropical region, and plants grow well. Ficus pumila is no exception, and we can harvest *Ficus pumila* L. all year round. Collect fresh, undried branches and leaves that are wrapped around trees in nature in the Motobu region. Boil 200 g of the leaves and branches together in 2 L of water to remove the branches and leaves to extract the ingredients. The heating temperature is 100 degrees and the heating time is 10 min. The water is used from the soil deposited by old corals in the Motobu region of Okinawa. This method is a traditional method that has been passed down orally for 600 years. Patients living in the Motobu region of Okinawa Prefecture took 300 mL of extract per day. The leaves are finely ground and extracted with a 50% aqueous solution of ethanol. The solvent is removed, fractionated by column chromatography, and then 1H NMR measurement is performed. Rutin, Apigenin, Luteolin, Quercetin, and Kaempferol were detected. Especially two hundred grams of *Ficus pumila* L. branch and leaf contain approximately 2.44 mg and 1.41 mg of Rutin and Apigenin, respectively. The polyphenol content in the extract given to the individuals was inspected by the Okinawa Prefectural Environmental Science Center, which is a registered inspection agency of the Minister of Health, Labour and Welfare of Japan under the Food Sanitation Law. The polyphenol content given to the individual is 0.15 g per day. The total amount of polyphenols contained in *Ficus pumila* L. was measured by the Folin–Ciocalteu method.

2.2. Data on the Patients

One hundred and twenty-eight rehabilitation patients developed diabetes within 1 year after COVID-19 infection (June–October 2022). In total, 128 were mild to moderate COVID-19 patients. There was no significant difference regarding the severity of COVID-19 between the patients. In total, 128 were given the antiviral drug molnupiravir. 128 had residual diabetes six months later. A total of 128 patients of the participants had not taken *Ficus pumila* L. extract before they were enrolled in the study. In total, 128 patients had not taken insulin treatment or oral hypoglycemic medication. Of the 128 patients who were still diabetic after 6 months, 59 (31 women and 28 men, mean age: 81 years) were from the Motobu region of Okinawa Prefecture and had taken *Ficus pumila* L. extract or at least 3 months after developing diabetes. Of the 128 subjects, 69 (35 women and 34 men, mean age: 80 years) were not from the Motobu region and were still diabetic after 6 months; in total, 69 had not taken *Ficus pumila* L. extract. Blood samples were collected at 07:30 a.m. after overnight fasting to measure fasting plasma glucose and fasting insulin levels. In total, 128 patients were diagnosed with diabetes mellitus with an early morning fasting blood glucose level of 126 mg/dL or more, a 75 g oral glucose tolerance test (OGTT) 2 h blood glucose level of 200 mg/dL or more, an hourly blood glucose level of 200 mg/dL or more, and an HbA1c (NGSP) of 6.5% or more. In addition, the immune-reactive insulin (IRI) level was 2.5 or higher, and insulin resistance was diagnosed. Prior to infection, the 128 patients had blood glucose, HbA1c, and IRI levels all within the baseline range, and did not develop diabetes. There was also no use of insulin.

2.3. Method and Equipment

A Homeostatic model assessment of β-cell function (HOMA-β) and that of insulin resistance (HOMA-IR) were used. Values were calculated using a HOMA calculator, which was available on the Diabetes Trials Unit website (https://www.rdm.ox.ac.uk/about/our-clinical-facilities-and-units/DTU/software/homa, accessed on 8 January 2025).

The equations for HOMA-β and HOMAIR are as follows.

$$\text{HOMA-}\beta = \text{Fasting insulin levels } (\mu\text{U/mL}) \times 360 \div (\text{Fasting blood glucose (mg/dL)} - 63)$$

$$\text{HOMA-IR} = \text{Fasting blood glucose (mg/dL)} \times \text{Fasting insulin levels } (\mu\text{U/mL})/405$$

HOMA-β is judged to be a decrease in insulin secretion capacity at 30% or less, and a marked decrease at 15% or less. HOMA-IR is judged to be insulin resistant at a time of 2.5 or higher. The HOMA-β and HOMA-IR were measured in 28 and 34 subjects.

Data are presented as means ± SD. p values were determined using Student's t-test. A p value < 0.05 was considered significant. SAS software version 9.2 (SAS Institute Inc., Cary, NC, USA) was used for statistical analysis.

3. Results

HOMA-β value significantly decreased after COVID-19 infection in the 59 subjects, (before; 59.4 ± 11.2 and after: 11.3 ± 7.8 $p < 0.05$, Figure 3a). However, HOMA-β significantly improved to 65.7 ± 13.1 after 3 months of *Ficus pumila* L. extract intake ($p < 0.05$, Figure 3a). The HOMA-IR before and after COVID-19 infection were 1.15 ± 0.28 and 4.96 ± 0.73 ($p < 0.05$, Figure 3b), respectively. The HOMA-IR value of the *Ficus pumila* L. extract ingested group was also significantly improved to 0.92 ± 0.31 after 3 months ($p < 0.05$, Figure 3b). On the other hand, the pre- and post-infection HOMA-β values of the 69 control subjects without *Ficus pumila* L. extract ingestion were 61.8 ± 12.4 and 13.5 ± 6.3 ($p < 0.05$, Figure 3c), respectively. The value further decreased to 11.9 ± 10.7 (Figure 3c). The HOMA-IR before and after infection were 0.97 ± 0.32 and 3.86 ± 0.41 ($p < 0.05$, Figure 3d), respectively. The value further increased to 3.72 ± 0.54 (Figure 3d). Results of normal people or people with diabetes who do not have COVID-19 and who are taking *Ficus pumila* L. extract have not been obtained.

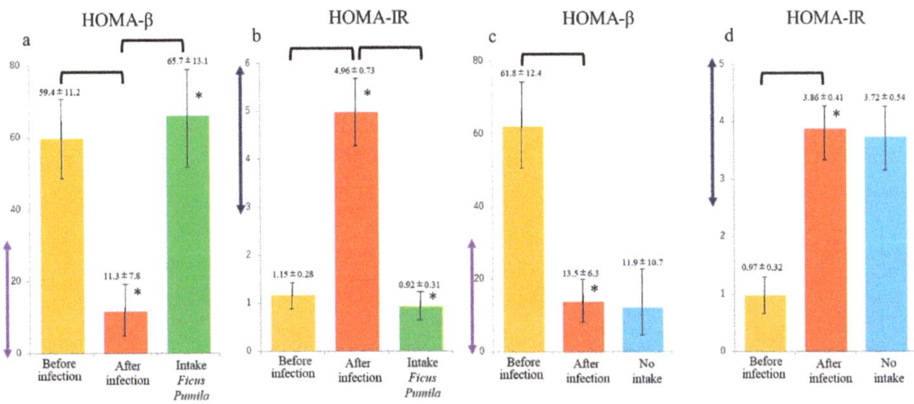

Figure 3. Results of HOMA-β and HOMA-IR evaluation. (**a**) Before COVID-19 infection, HOMA-β levels were within normal range. (orange box) HOMA-β levels decreased after infection (red box), but increased after consumption of *Ficus pumila* L. (green box). (**b**) Before COVID-19 infection, HOMA-IR levels were within normal range. (orange box). HOMA-IR evaluation after infection increased (red box), but decreased after ingestion of *Ficus pumila* L. (green box). (**c**) Before COVID-19 infection, HOMA-β levels were within normal range. (orange box) Post-infection HOMA-β levels decreased (red box) but continued to decrease. (blue box). (**d**) Before COVID-19 infection, HOMA-IR levels were within normal range. (orange box). Post-infection HOMA-IR levels increased (red box), but remained elevated. (blue box). Data are presented as average ± SD. * shows $p < 0.05$. HOMA-β levels: decreased insulin secretion capacity at 30% or less (violet two-way arrow). HOMA-IR levels: insulin resistance higher than 2.5 (purple two-way arrow).

4. Discussion

A patient with diabetes mellitus after COVID-19 infection died after acute pancreatitis and diabetic necrosis. Even mild or moderate COVID-19 infection can become serious if diabetes is later developed. If non-diabetic patients develop diabetes due to COVID-19 infection, the mechanism should be elucidated and cured. Therefore, we focused on the efficacy of *Ficus pumila* L. extract, which has been ingested in Okinawa as a folk remedy since ancient times. In the present study, *Ficus pumila* L. extract, ingested by patients who developed diabetes after COVID-19 infection, stimulated insulin secretion capacity and improved insulin resistance.

4.1. Pathogenesis of the Development of Diabetes Mellitus in Coronavirus Infection

Inhibition of Neuropilin 1 (NRP1), which is expressed in pancreatic tissue, has been reported to improve glucose tolerance in type 2 diabetes as well as in glucose intolerance after SARS-CoV2 infection [7–9]. Proteins such as ACE2 co-receptors NRP2 may also be responsible for worsening the COVID-19 course although many mechanisms associated with Angiotensin I-converting enzyme type 2 (ACE2) can lead to increased SARS-CoV-2 virulence in diabetes mellitus [10]. The SARS-CoV-2 proteins interact with targets such as the ACE2 receptor. In addition, SARS-CoV-2 can stimulate pathological intracellular signaling pathways by triggering NRP1. ACE2 may also be involved in reduced insulin secretion after SARS-CoV-2 infection. Consistently, high ACE2 expression in the islets of type 2 diabetes patients is reported to increase their susceptibility to SARS-CoV-2 infection, leading to impaired glucose metabolism [11]. The S-glycoprotein (Spike) of the SARS-CoV-2 forms a complex with the human transmembrane protein ACE2 during infection. ACE2 is a host receptor for SARS-CoV-2. Inhibiting the interaction between the envelope Spike of SARS-CoV-2 and ACE2 is a potential antiviral therapeutic approach, but little is known about how dietary compounds interact with ACE2.

In this study, *Ficus pumila* L. consumption also improved insulin resistance as indicated by HOMA-IR. Insulin resistance is closely related to the expression of glucose transport (GLUT) receptors on the cell surface of peripheral organs such as skeletal muscle. In particular, there is a correlation between the expression of GLUT4 and the level of insulin resistance [12]. Reduced GLUT4 expression is one of the causes of developing insulin resistance in type 2 diabetes [13]. It has been reported that ACE2 expression, a SARS-CoV-2 receptor, decreases with infection in peripheral tissues and this may lead to a decrease in GLUT4 expression, which ultimately develops insulin resistance [14,15]. SARS-CoV-2 also binds to ACE2 expressed in skeletal muscle tissues and induces inflammatory effects, cytokinesis, and muscle catabolism, damaging the musculoskeletal system [16]. Injury of skeletal muscle fibers by SARS-CoV-2 infection has also been reported to decrease the expression of GLUT4 [17].

4.2. Antioxidant Targets in the Treatment of COVID-19 and Complications

The polyphenol compounds inhibited 50% of virus–receptor binding interactions for NRP1 and ACE2, respectively. Polyphenol compounds more significantly interacted with the NRP1 receptor. Especially Quercetin was a compound with the highest exhibited interfering potential for selected target receptors [18]. Polyphenol is a known NRP1,2 inhibitor, and since *Ficus pumila* L. also contains polyphenols, it is possible that the action of polyphenol in *Ficus pumila* L. may have normalized insulin secretory capacity in patients presented in this study. Polyphenols, which are also the ingredients of *Ficus pumila* L., inhibit recombinant human ACE2 activity, which may prevent the development of type 2 diabetes [19]. Polyphenols are the major phytoconstituents that display antidiabetic activity by interacting with key protein molecules related to the MAPK and PI3K-AKT signaling pathways, thereby aiding in the treatment of type 2 diabetes mellitus.

4.3. Arguments Related to the Consequences of Treating Diabetes Post-COVID-19 with Antioxidant Therapy According to the Literature

Rutin and Quercetin inhibited rhACE2 activity. In particular, Quercetin was the most potent rhACE2 inhibitor among the polyphenols tested [20]. Quercetin and Rutin had remarkable antiviral potential against different viral infections. Rutin is an antiviral drug with high binding affinity to proteins SARS-CoV-2, SARS-CoV, and SARS-CoV-2 Spike protein [21]. It has been reported that SARS-CoV-2 infection decreases insulin expression in β-cells and further induces apoptosis of β-cells, resulting in decreased insulin secretory capacity [22]. Polyphenols are also thought to have protective effects on pancreatic β-cells [23] in Figure 4a. Rutin and Quercetin are promising polyphenols that showed great activity against diabetes and diabetes complications in vitro and in vivo, induced glucose uptake via increasing GLUT-4 expression and/or translocation through insulin signaling pathway, AMPK pathway or acting as partial PPAR-γ agonists [24]. The Apigenin, Luteolin, and Kaempferol increased the expressions of PPAR-γ and GLUT4; they induced GLUT4 translocation [25]. Treatment with Kaempferol 3-O-rutinoside resulted in the upregulation of insulin-dependent p-IRS, AKT, and AMPK signaling molecules, and stimulation of the GLUT4 translocation, which ultimately enhanced the glucose uptake in insulin-resistant skeletal muscle myotubes [26]. GLUT4, AKT2, and AMPK were docked with Quercetin and Kaempferol. Hyperglycaemia and insulin sensitivity via activation of AKT2 and AMPK were ameliorated, and the expression of GLUT4, AKT2, and AMPK, whose levels were reduced under diabetic conditions, increased [27]. Polyphenols increased mRNA expressions of GLUT4 in the pancreas and demonstrated a good anti-diabetic profile by improving insulin sensitivity and GLUT-4 translocation [28] in Figure 4b.

The pathological mechanism of developing diabetes, after COVID-19 infection, is still unclear [29,30]. Due to the limited number of cases of diabetes caused by COVID-19, opinions are still divided [31]. However, the results of this study suggest that at least the point of action of *Ficus pumila* L. may be involved in the development of diabetes after COVID-19 infection, and the results may contain important insights not only into the mechanism of diabetes development after COVID-19 infection but also for the treatment.

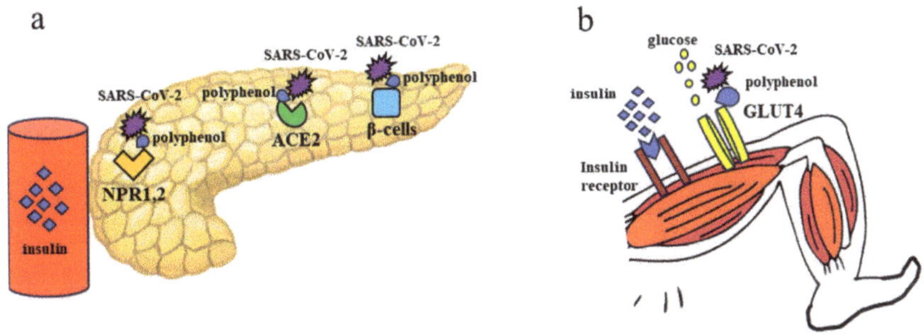

Figure 4. Pancreas and axial of femoral muscle. (**a**) Pancreas. Polyphenols protect the function of β-cells and inhibit Neuropilin 1, 2 (NPR1,2) and recombinant human ACE2 activity in pancreatic tissue infected with SARS-CoV-2. Insulin secretion deficiency improves, leading to increased secretion and increased amount of insulin in the blood. (**b**) Quadriceps femoris. Polyphenols stimulate GLUT4 expression, which is decreased by SARS-CoV-2 infection. Insulin and glucose bind to GLUT4 and are taken up by muscle cells. Insulin and glucose bind to GLUT4 and are taken up by muscle cells. Insulin resistance is improved, allowing insulin and glucose to be taken up into the muscles.

5. Conclusions

Ficus pumila L. extract can improve insulin secretory capacity and insulin resistance in post-COVID-19 infection-induced diabetes.

Author Contributions: Conceptualization, K.G.; methodology, K.G.; software, K.G.; validation, K.G.; formal analysis, K.G.; investigation, K.G.; resources, K.G. and T.H.; data curation, K.G. and K.S. (Kouichi Suzuki); writing—original draft preparation, K.G.; writing—review and editing, A.O. and T.S.; visualization, K.G.; supervision, S.T., Y.M. and K.S. (Kenjyu Shimomura). All authors have read and agreed to the published version of the manuscript.

Funding: This research received no external funding.

Institutional Review Board Statement: The study was conducted in accordance with the Declaration of Helsinki, and approved by the Institutional Review Board Ethics Review Board of Daido Central Hospital (no. 20, 1 September 2022) approved the study. All procedures were performed in accordance with the ethical standards of the committee responsible for human experimentation at Fukushima Medical University.

Informed Consent Statement: Written informed consent has been obtained from the patient(s) to publish this paper.

Data Availability Statement: The original contributions presented in this study are included in the article. Further inquiries can be directed to the corresponding author.

Acknowledgments: The authors would also like to thank the Okinawan patients for their participation in this study. This study was part of the Okinawa–Fukushima Obesity Project and Drug Research for Astatine-221 Targeted Alfa Therapy Project. Gonda, the corresponding author, participating in this project and practiced medicine in Okinawa Prefecture. *Ficus pumila* L. was named by Carl von Linne. The botanist Carl von Linne gave many scientific names to plants native to Japan. We pay tribute to botanist Carl von Linne.

Conflicts of Interest: The authors declare no conflicts of interest.

References

1. Xie, Y.; Al-Aly, Z. Risks and burdens of incident diabetes in long COVID: A cohort study. *Lancet Diabetes Endocrinol.* **2022**, *10*, 311–321. [CrossRef] [PubMed]
2. Wander, P.L.; Lowy, E.; Beste, L.A.; Tulloch-Palomino, L.; Korpak, A.; Peterson, A.C.; Kahn, S.E.; Boyko, E.J. The Incidence of Diabetes Among 2,777,768 Veterans With and Without Recent SARS-CoV-2 Infection. *Diabetes Care* **2022**, *45*, 782–788. [CrossRef]
3. Suzuki, K.; Gonda, K.; Kishimoto, Y.; Katsumoto, Y.; Takenoshita, S. Potential curing and beneficial effects of Ooitabi (*Ficus pumila* L.) on hypertension and dyslipidaemia in Okinawa. *J. Hum. Nutr. Diet.* **2021**, *34*, 395–401. [CrossRef] [PubMed]
4. Gonda, K.; Kanazawa, H.; Maeda, G.; Matayoshi, C.; Hirose, N.; Katsumoto, Y.; Kono, K.; Takenoshita, S. Ingestion of Okinawa Island Vegetables Increases IgA Levels and Prevents the Spread of Influenza RNA Viruses. *Nutrients* **2021**, *13*, 1773. [CrossRef] [PubMed]
5. Chen, J.; Mei, M.S.; Xu, Y.; Xiong, S.; Zhao, Y.; Liu, R.; Shi, S.; Wang, H.; Wang, S. The impact of the methyl esters of homogalacturonan on cellular uptake dependent hypoglycemic activity in IR-HepG2 cells. *Carbohydr. Polym.* **2022**, *293*, 119741. [CrossRef]
6. Qi, Z.-Y.; Zhao, J.-Y.; Lin, F.-J.; Zhou, W.-L.; Gan, R.-Y. Bioactive Compounds, Therapeutic Activities, and Applications of *Ficus pumila* L. *Agronomy* **2021**, *11*, 89. [CrossRef]
7. Wu, C.T.; Lidsky, P.V.; Xiao, Y.; Lee, I.T.; Cheng, R.; Nakayama, T.; Jiang, S.; Demeter, J.; Bevacqua, R.J.; Chang, C.A.; et al. SARS-CoV-2 infects human pancreatic β cells and elicits β cell impairment. *Cell Metab.* **2021**, *33*, 1565–1576. [CrossRef]
8. Ji, N.; Zhang, M.; Ren, L.; Wang, Y.; Hu, B.; Xiang, J.; Gong, Y.; Wu, C.; Qu, G.; Ding, W.; et al. SARS-CoV-2 in the pancreas and the impaired islet function in COVID-19 patients. *Emerg. Microbes Infect.* **2022**, *11*, 1115–1125. [CrossRef]
9. Costa, R.; Rodrigues, I.; Guardão, L.; Lima, J.Q.; Sousa, E.; Soares, R.; Negrão, R. Modulation of VEGF signaling in a mouse model of diabetes by xanthohumol and 8-prenylnaringenin: Unveiling the angiogenic paradox and metabolism interplay. *Mol. Nutr. Food Res.* **2017**, *61*, 201600488. [CrossRef] [PubMed]
10. Drzymała, A. The Functions of SARS-CoV-2 Receptors in Diabetes-Related Severe COVID-19. *Int. J. Mol. Sci.* **2024**, *25*, 9635. [CrossRef]
11. Fignani, D.; Pedace, E.; Licata, G.; Grieco, G.E.; Aiello, E.; de Luca, C.; Marselli, L.; Marchetti, P.; Sebastiani, G.; Dotta, F. Angiotensin I-converting enzyme type 2 expression is increased in pancreatic islets of type 2 diabetic donors. *Diabetes Metab. Res. Rev.* **2023**, *39*, e3696. [CrossRef] [PubMed]
12. Herman, R.; Kravos, N.A.; Jensterle, M.; Janež, A.; Dolžan, V. Metformin and Insulin Resistance: A Review of the Underlying Mechanisms behind Changes in GLUT4-Mediated Glucose Transport. *Int. J. Mol. Sci.* **2022**, *23*, 1264. [CrossRef] [PubMed]
13. van Gerwen, J.; Shun-Shion, A.S.; Fazakerley, D.J. Insulin signalling and GLUT4 trafficking in insulin resistance. *Biochem. Soc. Trans.* **2023**, *51*, 1057–1069. [CrossRef] [PubMed]
14. Govender, N.; Khaliq, O.P.; Moodley, J.; Naicker, T. Insulin resistance in COVID-19 and diabetes. *Prim. Care Diabetes.* **2021**, *15*, 629–634. [CrossRef]
15. Behera, J.; Ison, J.; Voor, M.J.; Tyagi, S.C.; Tyagi, N. Diabetic COVID-19 severity: Impaired glucose tolerance and pathologic bone loss. *Biochem. Biophys. Res. Commun.* **2022**, *620*, 180–187. [CrossRef]
16. Pescaru, C.C.; Marițescu, A.; Costin, E.O.; Trăilă, D.; Marc, M.S.; Trușculescu, A.A.; Pescaru, A.; Oancea, C.I. The Effects of COVID-19 on Skeletal Muscles, Muscle Fatigue and Rehabilitation Programs Outcomes. *Medicina* **2022**, *58*, 1199. [CrossRef]
17. Knudsen, J.R.; Persson, K.W.; Henriquez-Olguin, C.; Li, Z.; Di Leo, N.; Hesselager, S.A.; Raun, S.H.; Hingst, J.R.; Trouillon, R.; Wohlwend, M.; et al. Microtubule-mediated GLUT4 trafficking is disrupted in insulin-resistant skeletal muscle. *Elife* **2023**, *12* e83338. [CrossRef]
18. Suručić, R.; Radović Selgrad, J.; Kundaković-Vasović, T.; Lazović, B.; Travar, M.; Suručić, L.; Škrbić, R. In Silico and In Vitro Studies of Alchemilla viridiflora Rothm-Polyphenols' Potential for Inhibition of SARS-CoV-2 Internalization. *Molecules* **2022**, *27*, 5174. [CrossRef] [PubMed]
19. Guo, T.L.; Germolec, D.R.; Zheng, J.F.; Kooistra, L.; Auttachoat, W.; Smith, M.J.; White, K.L.; Elmore, S.A. Genistein protects female nonobese diabetic mice from developing type 1 diabetes when fed a soy- and alfalfa-free diet. *Toxicol. Pathol.* **2015**, *43*, 435–448. [CrossRef]
20. Liu, X.; Raghuvanshi, R.; Ceylan, F.D.; Bolling, B.W. Quercetin and Its Metabolites Inhibit Recombinant Human Angiotensin-Converting Enzyme 2 (ACE2) Activity. *J. Agric. Food Chem.* **2020**, *68*, 13982–13989. [CrossRef]
21. Rashid, Z.; Fatima, A.; Khan, A.; Matthew, J.; Yousaf, M.Z.; Nadeem, N.; Hasan, T.N.; Rehman, M.U.; Naqvi, S.S.; Khan, S.J. Drug repurposing: Identification of SARS-CoV-2 potential inhibitors by virtual screening and pharmacokinetics strategies. *J. Infect. Dev. Ctries.* **2024**, *18*, 520–531. [CrossRef]
22. Tang, X.; Uhl, S.; Zhang, T.; Xue, D.; Li, B.; Vandana, J.J.; Acklin, J.A.; Bonnycastle, L.L.; Narisu, N.; Erdos, M.R.; et al. SARS-CoV-2 infection induces beta cell transdifferentiation. *Cell Metab.* **2021**, *33*, 1577–1591. [CrossRef] [PubMed]

23. Saldanha, E.; Rao, S.; Adnan, M.; Pais, M.L.J.; Naik, T.S.; D'Cunha, R.; D'souza, R.; Baliga, M.S. Chapter 1—Polyphenols in the Prevention of Acute Pancreatitis in Preclinical Systems of Study: A Revisit. In *Polyphenols: Mechanisms of Action in Human Health and Disease*, 2nd ed.; Elsevier: Amsterdam, The Netherlands, 2018; pp. 3–9.
24. Akdad, M.; Ameziane, R.; Khallouki, F.; Bakri, Y.; Eddouks, M. Antidiabetic Phytocompounds Acting as Glucose Transport Stimulators. *Endocr. Metab. Immune Disord. Drug Targets* **2023**, *23*, 147–168. [PubMed]
25. Ortiz-Barragán, E.; Estrada-Soto, S.; Giacoman-Martínez, A.; Alarcón-Aguilar, F.J.; Fortis-Barrera, Á.; Marquina-Rodríguez, H.; Gaona-Tovar, E.; Lazzarini-Lechuga, R.; Suárez-Alonso, A.; Almanza-Pérez, J.C. Antihyperglycemic and Hypolipidemic Activities of Flavonoids Isolated from Smilax Dominguensis Mediated by Peroxisome Proliferator-Activated Receptors. *Pharmaceuticals* **2024**, *17*, 1451. [CrossRef]
26. Eddouks, M.; Akdad, M.; Ameziane, R.; Khallouki, F.; Bakri, Y. Kaempferol 3-O-rutinoside from Antidesma acidum Retz. Stimulates glucose uptake through SIRT1 induction followed by GLUT4 translocation in skeletal muscle L6 cells. *J. Ethnopharmacol.* **2023**, *301*, 115788.
27. Thabah, D.; Syiem, D.; Pakyntein, C.L.; Banerjee, S.; Kharshiing, C.E.; Bhattacharjee, A. Potentilla fulgens upregulate GLUT4, AMPK, AKT and insulin in alloxan-induced diabetic mice: An in vivo and in silico study. *Arch. Physiol. Biochem.* **2023**, *129*, 1071–1083. [CrossRef] [PubMed]
28. Asghar, A.; Sharif, A.; Awan, S.J.; Akhtar, B.; Akhtar, M.F.; Ali, S.; Shahnaz. Ficus johannis Boiss. leaves ethanolic extract ameliorate streptozotocin-induced diabetes in rats by upregulating the expressions of GCK, GLUT4, and IGF and downregulating G6P. *Environ. Sci. Pollut. Res. Int.* **2023**, *30*, 49108–49124. [CrossRef] [PubMed]
29. Gao, J.; Cao, C.; Shi, M.; Hong, S.; Guo, S.; Li, J.; Liang, T.; Song, P.; Xu, R.; Li, N. Kaempferol inhibits SARS-CoV-2 invasion by impairing heptad repeats-mediated viral fusion. *Phytomedicine* **2023**, *118*, 154942. [CrossRef]
30. Ożarowski, M.; Karpiński, T.M. The Effects of Propolis on Viral Respiratory Diseases. *Molecules* **2023**, *28*, 359. [CrossRef]
31. Zarei, A.; Ramazani, A.; Rezaei, A.; Moradi, S. Screening of honey bee pollen constituents against COVID-19: An emerging hot spot in targeting SARS-CoV-2-ACE-2 interaction. *Nat. Prod. Res.* **2023**, *37*, 974–980. [CrossRef]

nutrients

MDPI

Article

Antihypertensive Effects of *Lindera erythrocarpa* Makino via NO/cGMP Pathway and Ca^{2+} and K^+ Channels

Sujin Shin [1], Junkyu Park [2], Ho-Young Choi [3], Youngmin Bu [3] and Kyungjin Lee [3,*]

1 Department of Korean Medicine, Graduate School, Kyung Hee University, Seoul 02447, Republic of Korea; sjshin04@khu.ac.kr
2 Department of Science in Korean Medicine, Graduate School, Kyung Hee University, Seoul 02447, Republic of Korea; ojeoksan@khu.ac.kr
3 Department of Herbal Pharmacology, College of Korean Medicine, Kyung Hee University, Seoul 02447, Republic of Korea; hychoi@khu.ac.kr (H.-Y.C.); ymbu@khu.ac.kr (Y.B.)
* Correspondence: niceday@khu.ac.kr

Abstract: Studies have demonstrated the therapeutic effects of *Lindera* plants. This study was undertaken to reveal the antihypertensive properties of *Lindera erythrocarpa* leaf ethanolic extract (LEL). Aorta segments of Sprague–Dawley rats were used to study the vasodilatory effect of LEL, and the mechanisms involved were evaluated by treating specific inhibitors or activators that affect the contractility of blood vessels. Our results revealed that LEL promotes a vasorelaxant effect through the nitric oxide/cyclic guanosine 3′,5′-monophosphate pathway, blocking the Ca^{2+} channels, opening the K^+ channels, and inhibiting the vasoconstrictive action of angiotensin II. In addition, the effects of LEL on blood pressure were investigated in spontaneously hypertensive rats by the tail-cuff method. LEL (300 or 1000 mg/kg) was orally administered to the rats, and 1000 mg/kg of LEL significantly lowered the blood pressure. Systolic blood pressure decreased by $-20.06 \pm 4.87\%$, and diastolic blood pressure also lowered by $-30.58 \pm 5.92\%$ at 4 h in the 1000 mg/kg LEL group. Overall, our results suggest that LEL may be useful to treat hypertensive diseases, considering its vasorelaxing and hypotensive effects.

Keywords: *Lindera erythrocarpa*; blood pressure; hypertension; hypotensive effect; spontaneously hypertensive rat; vasorelaxant; endothelium; NO/cGMP pathway; angiotensin II

1. Introduction

Cardiovascular diseases (CVDs) are major noncommunicable diseases (NCDs) and account for approximately 50% of the NCD-related deaths [1]. Among the risk factors for CVDs, hypertension is one of the most compelling indicators of a causal relationship and is associated with a higher frequency of exposure [2]. Maintaining normal blood pressure is crucial; however, hypertension is often deemed an inevitable part of aging, with a prevalence of 60–75% in older adults (≥60 years) [3,4]. With the rapidly aging population, the prevalence of hypertension is anticipated to escalate further [5]. However, a recent study found that more than half of the patients with hypertension in the United States have uncontrolled blood pressure [6]. Therefore, new therapeutic and preventive strategies are needed to manage patients with high blood pressure.

Medicinal plants have emerged as potential agents for managing CVDs and have been proven to be beneficial in reducing cardiovascular risk factors [7]. The therapeutic potential of plants is mainly attributed to their bioactive compounds, including polyphenols, dietary fibers, and carotenoids [8,9]. In particular, plants and their natural compounds have shown hypotensive effects by promoting vasorelaxation through various mechanisms, which include stimulating the nitric oxide (NO)/cyclic guanosine 3′,5′-monophosphate (cGMP) signaling pathway, inhibiting angiotensin-converting enzymes, or blocking the Ca^{2+} channels [10,11]. Additionally, several commercially available drugs for CVDs, including ephedrine, digitoxin, and salicin, originate from plants [12]. Although many plants and their natural compounds have demonstrated benefits in managing hypertension, their specific mechanisms of action remain unknown. Therefore, further research is required to gain a deeper understanding of their inherent complexities.

The genus *Lindera* holds economic significance due to its utilization in teas, spices, and fragrances. Furthermore, *Lindera* exhibits notable medicinal and therapeutic effects attributed to its diverse pharmacological properties [13,14]. Studies have demonstrated the anti-hypertensive effects of *Lindera* species [15,16]. *L. erythrocarpa* (LE) has been used as an herbal remedy for treating digestive disorders, alleviating thirst, and managing pain [17]. Recent studies have revealed various components of LE, such as linderone, lucidone, kanakuziol, camphene, and limonene, showcasing their diverse effects including anti-inflammatory, anticancer, and antifungal activities [18]. However, no studies have investigated the anti-hypertensive effects of LE. Therefore, this study investigated the vascular effects of LE leaf 50% ethanol extract (LEL) on aorta rings of Sprague–Dawley (SD) rats under various experimental conditions. In addition, the hypotensive effect of LEL oral administration in spontaneously hypertensive rats (SHRs) was assessed.

2. Materials and Methods

2.1. Preparation of the Extract

LEL samples were collected from Seogwipo-si, Jeju, Republic of Korea, in June 2023 and authenticated by Prof. Ho-Young Choi in the Department of Herbal Pharmacology, College of Korean Medicine, Kyung Hee University. The LEL samples were deposited at the College of Korean Medicine, Kyung Hee University, Seoul, Republic of Korea. Dried and grinded LEL samples were extracted by boiling them with 50% ethanol for 2 h at 70 ± 2 °C. After filtration, the extract was freeze-dried. The extract yield of LEL was 18.57% (extract yield = weight of the final freeze-dried extract/weight of the dried sample $\times$ 100).

2.2. Animals

Male SD rats (6–7 weeks old) were provided by Daehan Bio Link (Eumseong-gun, Republic of Korea), and male SHRs (16–17 weeks old) were provided by SLC, Inc. (Shizuoka, Japan). Animals were housed under standard laboratory conditions with free access to food and tap water. All experimental protocols were approved by the Institutional Animal Care and Use Committee of Kyung Hee University (approval number: KHSASP-23-506 on 17 November 2023).

2.3. Chemicals and Solution Preparation

Dimethyl sulfoxide (DMSO) was obtained from Junsei (Tokyo, Japan). Phenylephrine (PE), acetylcholine (ACh), indomethacin, methylene blue (MB), ethyleneglycol-bis(2-aminoethylether)-N,N,N,′N′-tetraacetic acid (EGTA), Bay K8644, and angiotensin II were provided by Sigma Aldrich (St. Louis, MA, USA). N^G-nitro-L-arginine methyl ester (L-NAME), 4-aminopyridine (4-AP), and tetraethylammonium (TEA) were purchased from Wako Pure Chemical Industries (Osaka, Japan). 1H-[1,2,4] oxadiazolo [4,3-a]quinoxalin-1-one (ODQ) was purchased from the Tokyo Chemical Industry (Tokyo, Japan). All other reagents were provided by Daejeong Chemical & Gold (Siheung-si, Republic of Korea).

The composition of the Krebs Henseleit (KH) solution, mM, was as follows: NaCl, 118; KCl, 4.7; KH_2PO_4, 1.2; $MgSO_4$, 1.2; $CaCl_2$, 2.5; $NaHCO_3$, 25; and glucose, 11.1.

2.4. Ex Vivo Vasorelaxant Evaluation

2.4.1. General Experimental Procedures

The vasodilatory effect was evaluated following the established methods [19]. Briefly, the SD rats were sacrificed with urethane (1.2 g/kg, intraperitoneal injection). The thoracic aorta was extracted and was cleaned of the adjacent and connective tissue. Multiple aortic rings from one SD rat were cut to the same length and assigned to either the control or experimental group to minimize intergroup differences. Each ring was considered an experimental unit. Rings were mounted between hooks with a tension of 1.0 g in glass chambers containing KH solution bubbled with an O_2/CO_2 (95:5%) mixture and maintained at 37 °C. According to reliable statistics and animal ethics principles, we set the sample size to at least four per group, as described previously [20].

2.4.2. Role of Endothelium in LEL-Induced Vasorelaxant Activity

The endothelium-intact rings were assessed by relaxation (>85%) to ACh (10 μM) in the rings constricted with PE (1 μM). To process the endothelium-removed rings, the intimal surface of the artery was mechanically removed by rubbing with a smooth wooden stick. The endothelium-removed rings were assessed by relaxation (<10%) to ACh (10 μM). After confirming the endothelium, the rings were induced contraction by PE (1 μM). Following the attainment of the maximum blood vessel constriction by PE, the cumulative concentrations of LEL dissolved in DMSO were applied to KH buffer in the glass chamber containing endothelium-intact or endothelium-removed aorta.

2.4.3. Role of NO Synthase and Cyclooxygenase (COX) in LEL-Induced Vasorelaxant Activity

The thoracic aortic rings were incubated with L-NAME (an NO synthase inhibitor, 100 μM) or indomethacin (a COX inhibitor, 10 μM) for 20 min. After incubation, constriction of the rings was induced by PE (1 μM). Following the attainment of the maximum blood vessel contraction by PE, the cumulative concentrations of LEL were applied (0.5, 1, 2, 5, and 10 μg/mL).

2.4.4. Role of Soluble Guanylate Cyclase (sGC) and cGMP in LEL-Induced Vasorelaxant Activity

ODQ (an sGC inhibitor, 10 μM) or MB (a cGMP inhibitor, 10 μM) were applied to the aortic rings and incubated for 20 min. After incubation, contraction of the rings was induced by PE (1 μM). Following the attainment of the maximum blood vessel constriction by PE, the cumulative concentrations of LEL were applied (0.5, 1, 2, 5, and 10 μg/mL).

2.4.5. Effect of LEL on Ca^{2+} Influx through Ca^{2+} Channels

The aortic rings were stabilized in a Ca^{2+}-free KH solution with EGTA (1 mM). They were treated with LEL (100, 200, 500, and 1000 μg/mL) for 20 min and, subsequently, PE (1 μM) for 20 min. After incubation, the cumulative concentrations of $CaCl_2$ were applied.

2.4.6. Effect of LEL on Rings Constricted by Bay K8644

Rings were treated with LEL (1000 μg/mL) for 20 min. After incubation, Bay K8644 solution (L-type Ca^{2+} channel agonist, 10 μM) was introduced in each chamber.

2.4.7. Role of K^+ Channels in LEL-Induced Vasorelaxant Activity

$BaCl_2$ (inward rectifier K^+ channel blocker, 10 μM), 4-AP (voltage-dependent K^+ channel blocker, 1 mM) or TEA (large-conductance Ca^{2+}-activated K^+ channel blocker, 1 mM) were applied to the aortic rings and left to incubate for 20 min. Then, contraction of the rings was induced by PE (1 μM). Following the attainment of the maximum blood vessel contraction by PE, the cumulative concentrations of LEL were applied (0.5, 1, 2, 5, and 10 μg/mL).

2.4.8. Effect of LEL on Rings Constricted by Angiotensin II

The rings were treated with LEL (10 μg/mL) for 20 min. After incubation, angiotensin II (10^{-9}–10^{-6} M) was applied to each chamber.

2.5. Blood Pressure Measurement

SHRs were acclimated by measuring the blood pressure once a day for 1 week before the experiment. SHRs with systolic blood pressure (SBP) < 190 mmHg and diastolic blood pressure (DBP) < 140 mmHg were excluded from the study. Eighteen SHRs were randomly allocated into three groups for oral administration as follows: the control group (orally administered distilled water) and LEL groups at two different levels (orally administered 300 mg/kg and 1000 mg/kg of body weight dissolved in distilled water). Blood pressure was measured as previously described [19]. To minimize potential confounders, the blood pressure of one or two rats per group was measured simultaneously. The control group rats whose blood pressure was not maintained (difference of >20% from that measured before administration) were excluded from the analysis.

2.6. Statistical Analysis

Statistical analyses were performed using multiple unpaired *t*-tests and two-way analysis of variance with multiple comparisons (simple effects within rows), followed by Dunnett's post hoc test. Differences between the experimental and control groups were evaluated at the same concentrations or times. GraphPad Prism software version 9 (San Diego, CA, USA) was used for statistical procedures. In all the analyses, $p < 0.05$ was considered significant.

3. Results

3.1. Role of Endothelium in LEL-Induced Vasorelaxant Activity

LEL significantly relaxed the endothelium-intact aorta compared with the control in a dose-dependent manner, and the E_{max} value was 73.07 ± 5.50% at 10 μg/mL (Figure 1A,B). LEL also significantly relaxed the endothelium-absent rings, and the E_{max} value was 97.29 ± 0.39% at 1000 μg/mL (Figure 1C,D).

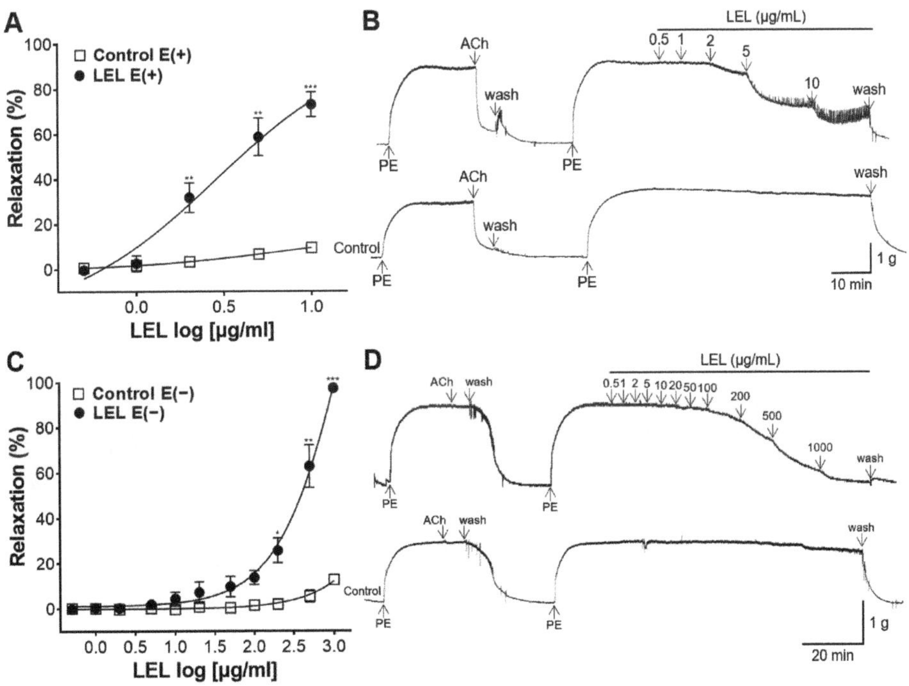

Figure 1. Effect of *Lindera erythrocarpa* leaf 50% ethanol extract (LEL) on endothelium-intact [E(+)] or endothelium-absent [E(−)] aorta, which underwent induced constriction with phenylephrine (PE, 1 μM). To confirm the endothelium, relaxation of pre-constricted aortas was induced by acetylcholine (ACh, 10 μM). (**A**,**C**) Relaxation response to LEL and (**B**,**D**) representative tracing. Data shown are the mean ± standard error of the mean (SEM) (n = 5). * $p < 0.05$, ** $p < 0.01$, *** $p < 0.001$ vs. control.

3.2. Role of NO Synthase and COX in LEL-Induced Vasorelaxant Activity

To elucidate the involvement of NO synthase and COX in LEL-induced relaxation, the aortic rings were incubated with L-NAME, a NO synthase inhibitor, or indomethacin, a COX inhibitor. LEL treatment with the incubation of L-NAME resulted in the reduced relaxation of the rings contracted by PE compared to the control; however, incubation with indomethacin did not reveal any significant effects on LEL-induced vasorelaxation (Figure 2).

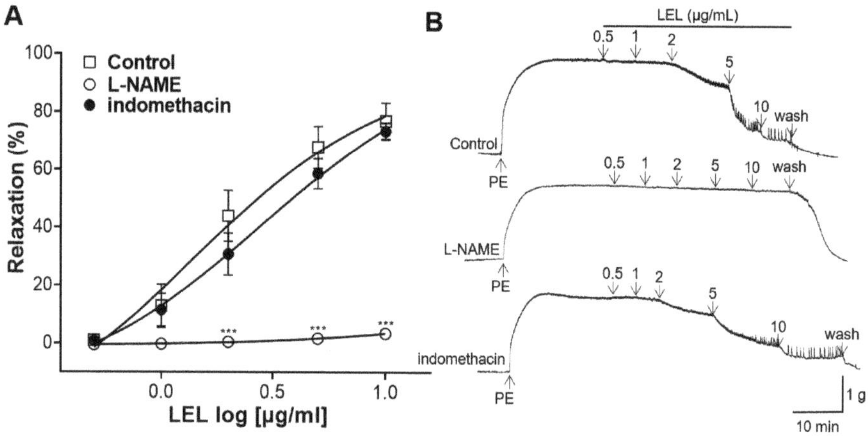

Figure 2. Effect of LEL on aortic rings which underwent induced constriction by PE (1 μM) without (Control) or with the incubation of L-NAME (100 μM) or indomethacin (10 μM). (**A**) Relaxation response to LEL and (**B**) representative tracing. Data shown are the mean ± SEM (n = 5–6). *** $p < 0.001$ vs. control.

3.3. Role of sGC and cGMP in LEL-Induced Vasorelaxant Activity

To determine the role of sGC and cGMP in LEL-induced vasorelaxant activity, the rings were incubated with ODQ, an sGC inhibitor, or MB, a cGMP inhibitor. LEL resulted in a significantly reduced relaxation of aortic rings in the presence of ODQ and MB (Figure 3).

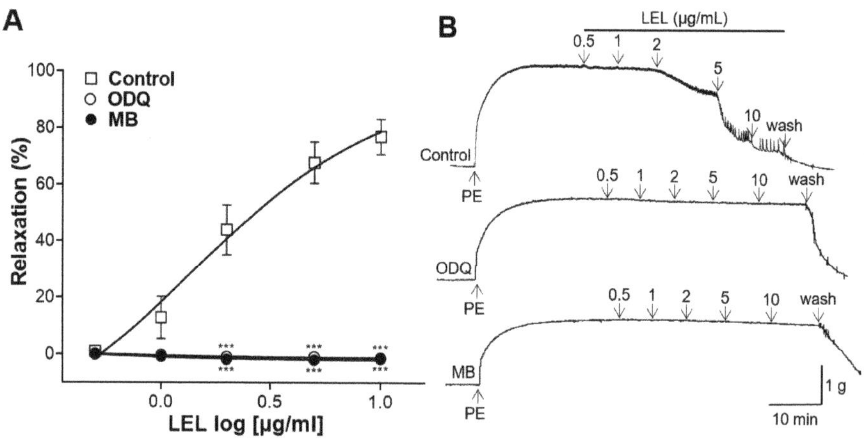

Figure 3. Effect of LEL on aortic rings with induced contraction by PE (1 μM), without (Control) or with the incubation of ODQ (10 μM) or MB (10 μM). (**A**) Relaxation response to LEL and (**B**) representative tracing. Data shown are the mean ± SEM (n = 5–6). *** $p < 0.001$ vs. control.

3.4. Effect of LEL on Ca^{2+} Influx

To elucidate the effect of LEL on Ca^{2+} influx via Ca^{2+} channels, the rings were constricted by $CaCl_2$. LEL (200, 500, and 1000 μg/mL) significantly reduced the contraction of aortic rings. The maximal contractions by $CaCl_2$ (10 mM) were 1.93 ± 0.11 g, 1.67 ± 0.27 g, 0.99 ± 0.10 g, 0.35 ± 0.12 g, and −0.18 ± 0.05 g in the absence and presence of LEL (100, 200, 500, and 1000 μg/mL), respectively (Figure 4).

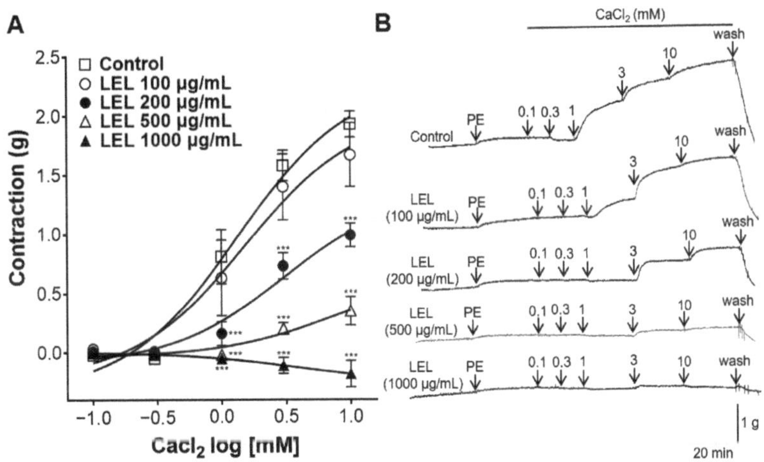

Figure 4. Effect of LEL on Ca^{2+} influx in the thoracic aorta. The rings were treated with PE (1 μM) before the constriction caused by $CaCl_2$. (**A**) Contraction response to $CaCl_2$ and (**B**) representative tracing. Data shown are the mean ± SEM (n = 4–6). *** $p < 0.001$ vs. control.

To investigate whether LEL has an inhibitory effect on L-type Ca^{2+} channels, the rings were constricted using Bay K8644 (an L-type Ca^{2+} channel agonist) in the rings incubated with or without LEL. Rings incubated with LEL (1000 μg/mL) showed a significant inhibitory effect on the contractions by Bay K 8644 (Figure 5).

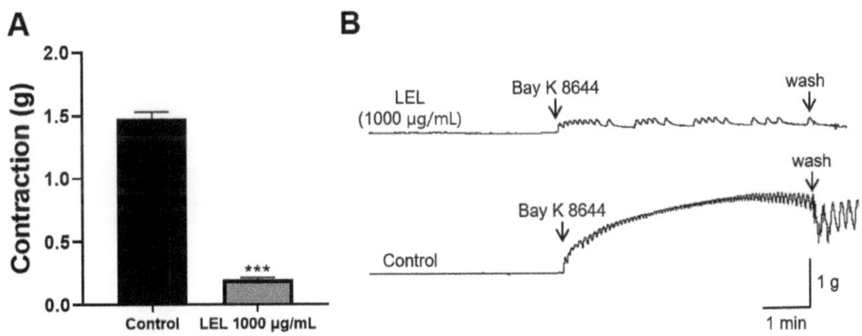

Figure 5. Effect of LEL on Ca^{2+} influx via L-type Ca^{2+} channel. LEL were applied to the rings (1000 μg/mL) before inducing contractions using Bay K8644 (10 μM). (**A**) Contraction response by Bay K8644 and (**B**) representative tracing. Data are presented as mean ± SEM (n = 5). *** $p < 0.001$ vs. control.

3.5. Role of K^+ Channels in LEL-Induced Vasorelaxant Activity

One of the following were applied to the aortic rings: inward rectifier K^+ channel blocker, $BaCl_2$, voltage-dependent K^+ channel blocker, 4-AP, or large-conductance Ca^{2+}-activated K^+ channel blocker, TEA. LEL resulted in the reduced relaxation of the aortic rings, which had undergone an induced contraction by PE, with the pre-incubation of 4-AP and TEA when compared to the control; however, the incubation with $BaCl_2$ showed no significant effects on the LEL-induced vasorelaxant activity in aortic rings contracted with PE (Figure 6).

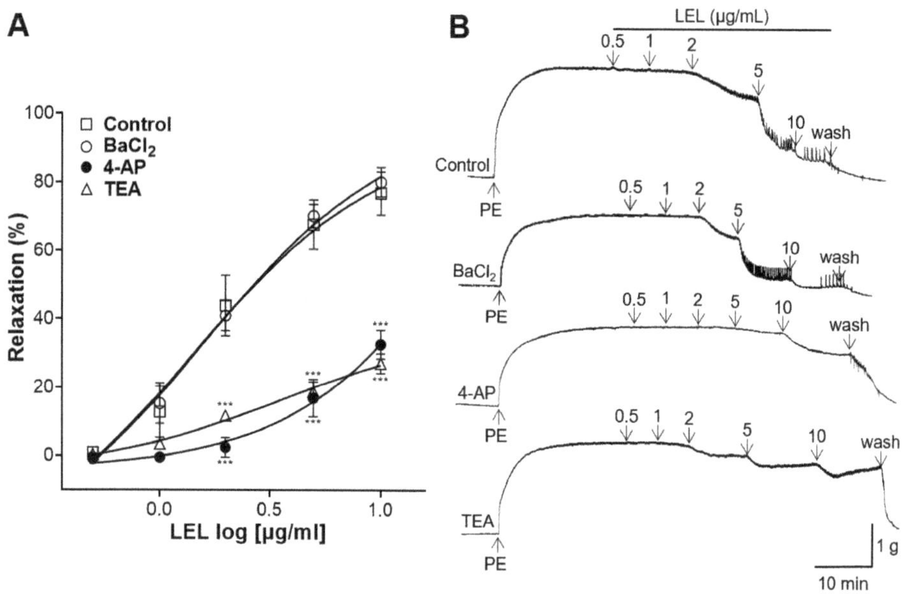

Figure 6. Effect of LEL on aortic rings with induced contraction by PE (1 μM) without (Control) or with the incubation of $BaCl_2$ (10 μM), 4-AP (1 mM), or TEA (1 mM). (**A**) Relaxation response to LEL and (**B**) representative tracing. Data shown are the mean ± SEM (n =5–6). *** $p < 0.001$ vs. control.

3.6. Effect of LEL on Rings Constricted by Angiotensin II

We assessed whether LEL inhibited the constrictive action of angiotensin II in thoracic aortic rings. The cumulative application of angiotensin II induced concentration-dependent contractions, and LEL (10 μg/mL) significantly attenuated these contractions (Figure 7). The maximal contractions by angiotensin II (10^{-6} M) of the aortic rings incubated without or with LEL were 1.29 ± 0.08 g and 0.79 ± 0.10 g, respectively.

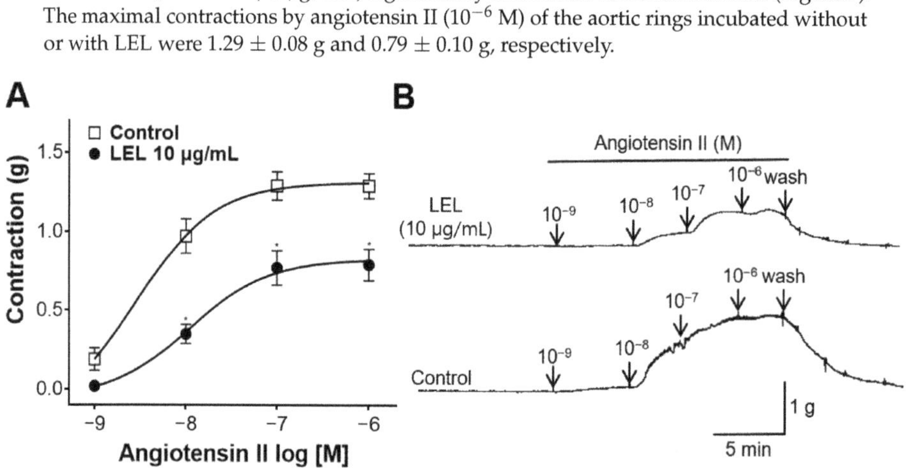

Figure 7. Effect of LEL on rings constricted by angiotensin II. (**A**) Contraction response to angiotensin II and (**B**) representative tracing. Data shown are the mean ± SEM (n = 4–5). * $p < 0.05$ vs. control.

3.7. Hypotensive Effect of LEL

The blood pressure after the oral administration of LEL to the SHRs are shown in Figure 8. 1000 mg/kg of LEL promoted a marked hypotensive effect in the SHRs compared to the control. The lowest was measured 4 h after the administration of 300 and 1000 mg/kg LEL, respectively. The SBP and DBP were reduced by $-9.34 \pm 2.86\%$ and $-15.19 \pm 3.92\%$, respectively, in the LEL 300 mg/kg group at 4 h after administration. However, there was no significant difference with the control group. The SBP and DBP were reduced by $-20.06 \pm 4.87\%$ and $-30.58 \pm 5.92\%$, respectively, in the LEL 1000 mg/kg group at 4 h after administration. The mean arterial blood pressure (MBP) also reduced significantly by $-24.54 \pm 5.28\%$ in the LEL 1000 mg/kg group at 4 h.

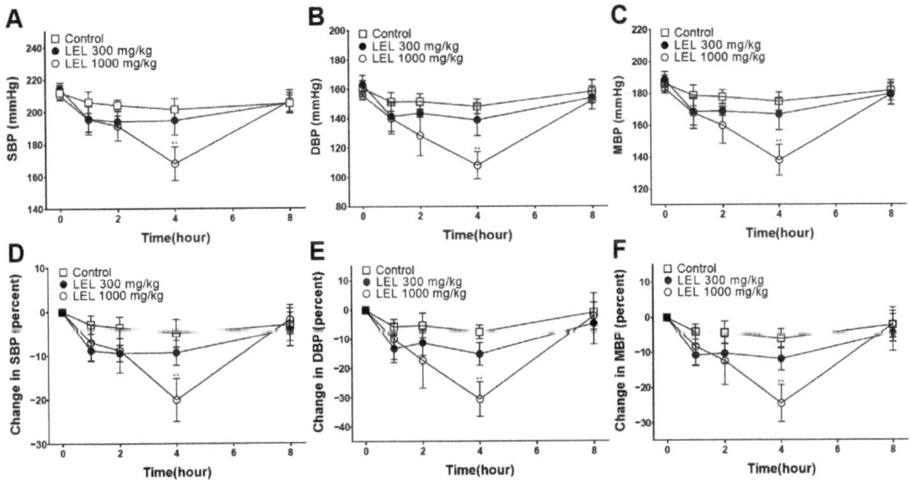

Figure 8. The effect of LEL on blood pressure. (**A**) SBP, (**B**) DBP, (**C**) MBP, (**D**) percent changes in SBP, (**E**) percent changes in DBP and (**F**) percent changes in MBP. Data shown are the mean ± SEM (n = 5). ** $p < 0.01$ vs. control.

4. Discussion

The effects of LEL on isolated aorta were investigated in this study. The cumulative administration of LEL promoted vasorelaxant activity of endothelium-intact and endothelium-absent rings in a dose-dependent manner. LEL induced a significant vasodilator effect with an E_{max} value of $73.07 \pm 5.50\%$ at 10 μg/mL in the endothelium-intact rings and $97.29 \pm 0.39\%$ at 1000 μg/mL in the endothelium-denuded rings. Our results indicate that the vascular relaxing effect of LEL is related to both the endothelium-dependent and endothelium-independent pathways. In addition, our results show that the vasodilatory effect of LEL acts primarily through an endothelium-dependent mechanism at relatively low doses, whereas at high concentrations, an endothelium-independent mechanism also acts.

After confirming the vasorelaxant effect of LEL, the endothelium-dependent mechanism in the vasorelaxant effects involved was investigated. The vascular endothelial cells are the primary regulators of vascular tone by various vasoactive agents, such as NO, prostacyclin (PGI_2), or endothelin-1 [21]. The major endothelial-derived vasodilator substances are NO and PGI_2 [21]. NO is a vasodilator that produces its effects mainly through the activation of sGC, which in turn promotes cGMP synthesis in VSMCs [22]. PGI_2, produced by COX, induces vasodilation and activates adenylate cyclase, which generates cyclic adenosine monophosphate (cAMP) [23]. Increased cGMP or cAMP levels lead to the relaxation of VSMCs and subsequent vasodilation [24]. To reveal the role of NO and PGI_2 in LEL-induced vasorelaxant activity, the aortic rings were incubated with L-NAME (an NO synthase inhibitor) or indomethacin (a COX inhibitor). Our results revealed that L-NAME treatment decreases the relaxation of the aortic rings; however, incubation with indomethacin did not display any significant effects on LEL-induced relaxation. To further elucidate the NO-related mechanisms related with the vasorelaxant effects of LEL, the rings were incubated with ODQ (an sGC inhibitor) or MB (a cGMP inhibitor). Our results showed that ODQ and MB pretreatment resulted in decreased relaxation compared to that of the control. Thus, our study shows that the mechanism underlying LEL-induced vasorelaxation involves the NO–sGC–cGMP pathway but is independent of PGI_2.

In VSMCs, contractions are primarily controlled by the intracellular concentration of Ca^{2+}, which activates and phosphorylates myosin light chain kinase, thereby enabling myosin to interact with actin [25]. Therefore, vasorelaxation in VSMCs can be achieved by reducing the intracellular Ca^{2+} concentration, inhibiting Ca^{2+} influx, promoting Ca^{2+} efflux, or increasing the uptake of Ca^{2+} into intracellular stores [26]. In the present study, we assessed the inhibitory effects of LEL on Ca^{2+} influx through Ca^{2+} channels. Aortic segments were pre-incubated with PE before treatment with $CaCl_2$ (0.1, 0.3, 1, 3, or 10 mM). LEL (200, 500, and 1000 μg/mL) significantly decreased Ca^{2+}-induced aortic ring constriction. PE-induced contraction involves various Ca^{2+} channels, such as L-type voltage-gated, receptor-operated, and store-operated Ca^{2+} channels [27]. Therefore, our study indicated that LEL can block the Ca^{2+} channels at high concentrations. LEL at concentrations of 100 μg/mL did not show a significant effect of blocking Ca^{2+} influx compared to the control group, and a significant inhibitory effect of LEL on Ca^{2+} influx was observed with doses $\geq$ 200 μg/mL (Figure 4). When the aortic rings were absent from the endothelium, significant vasorelaxation by LEL was observed with doses $\geq$ 200 μg/mL (Figure 1). Therefore, our study suggests that the Ca^{2+} channel-blocking effect of LEL is independent of the endothelium.

Among the various Ca^{2+} channels, L-type Ca^{2+} channels are crucial for initiating and maintaining VSMC contraction [28]. Additionally, owing to their wide distribution throughout the cardiovascular system, they are major pharmacological targets in treating hypertension and CVDs [29]. The inhibitory effects of LEL on L-type Ca^{2+} channels were investigated using Bay K8644, an L-type Ca^{2+} channel agonist. LEL (1000 μg/mL) exhibited a significant effect in inhibiting the contraction induced by Bay K8644. Therefore, our results indicate that LEL has an inhibitory effect on L-type Ca^{2+} channels.

The activation of K^+ channels is a key mechanism in achieving blood vessel relaxation, facilitating increased blood flow and decreased vascular resistance [30]. Several K^+ channels are related in this process, including inward rectifier K^+ channels, voltage-dependent K^+ channels, and large-conductance Ca^{2+}-activated K^+ channels [31]. The activation of these K^+ channels allows for the efflux of K^+ out of VSMCs and induces a hyperpolarization of the cell membrane and a reduction in the activity of Ca^{2+} channels, leading to reduced vasocontraction and thereby promoting relaxation [32]. Additional experiments were undertaken to elucidate the involvement of K^+ channels in LEL's vasorelaxant effects. Aortic rings were incubated with 4-AP (a voltage-dependent K^+ channel blocker), TEA (a large-conductance Ca^{2+}-activated K^+ channel blocker), or $BaCl_2$ (an inward rectifier K^+ channel blocker). Our results showed that 4-AP and TEA treatment resulted in reduced relaxation of the aortic rings compared to the control; however, incubation with $BaCl_2$ did not exert any significant effects on LEL-induced vasorelaxation. Therefore, our study suggests that the mechanism of LEL-induced vasorelaxation involves K^+ channels, particularly voltage-dependent and large-conductance Ca^{2+}-activated K^+ channels.

The role of angiotensin II was investigated to further explore the vasorelaxant effects of LEL. Angiotensin II, the major peptide in the renin–angiotensin system, is a potent vasoconstrictor that increases resistance of blood vessels and blood pressure [33]. The acute stimulation of angiotensin II induces the immediate vasoconstriction by increasing the intracellular Ca^{2+} concentration [33]. In our experiments, LEL-treated aortic rings showed significantly attenuated angiotensin II-induced contractions, indicating that LEL inhibited the constrictive action of angiotensin II.

Finally, the effect of LEL on blood pressure in the SHRs was investigated. The SHRs represent an established genetic model of hypertension developed by selective breeding which naturally exhibit high blood pressure and are similar in the development of essential hypertension with humans [34]. SHRs are useful for evaluating the effectiveness of antihypertensive drugs or interventions because of their predictable hypertensive phenotypes and similar responses to antihypertensive agents [35]. In our study, the oral administration of 1000 mg/kg LEL showed a significant hypotensive effect in the SHRs compared to the control. The lowest reduction rates in SBP and DBP ($-20.06 \pm 4.87\%$ and $-30.58 \pm 5.92\%$, respectively) were measured 4 h after administration in the LEL 1000 mg/kg group. Moreover, MBP showed the highest rate of decrease by $-24.54 \pm 5.28\%$ in the LEL 1000 mg/kg group at 4 h. Our results provide preliminary evidence that LEL alleviates hypertension. Adverse effects, such as sudden death or weight loss >20%, were not observed following administration. Further research, including long-term administration and toxicity testing, is warranted to validate the use of LEL in hypertension treatment.

Plants and their natural compounds have shown potential in the treatment of hypertension through various mechanisms [36]. Our study demonstrated that LEL exhibits a vasorelaxant effect through the NO/cGMP pathway, blocking Ca^{2+} channels, activating K^+ channels, and inhibits the constrictive action of angiotensin II. Blood pressure is regulated by the tone of the blood vessels, and relaxation of VSMCs leads to the dilation of the vessels and a reduction in the blood pressure [31]. This study demonstrated the vasodilatory properties and mechanisms of action of LEL in isolated rat thoracic aortas. The thoracic aorta of rats is the most commonly used model for studying vasodilation effects because of its accessibility and the ability to investigate mechanisms related to the endothelium and VSMCs [37]. However, considering that resistant arteries are key elements of vascular resistance and blood pressure, additional experiments are required to elucidate the vasorelaxant effects of LEL on smaller arteries [38]. In addition, LEL resulted in the reduction in blood pressure in the SHRs, which are an established model of essential hypertension. Overall, LEL may be a valuable source for the treatment of hypertensive diseases. In particular, plant leaves are easily accessible and have a history of usage in traditional medicine; therefore, LEL could be an effective and affordable alternative for treating hypertension [39]. Three marker compounds, methyl lucidone, methyl linderone, and kanakugiol, have been identified as the major contributors to the therapeutic effects of LE [40]. However, this study did not analyze the components of LEL. Therefore, further research is required to identify the active components of LEL for an enhanced understanding and potential commercial utilization.

5. Conclusions

This study demonstrated the anti-hypertensive properties of LEL. LEL exhibits a vasorelaxant effect through both endothelium-dependent and endothelium-independent mechanisms. The related mechanisms include the activation of NO–sGC–cGMP pathway, blocking the Ca^{2+} influx, opening K^+ channels, or inhibiting the angiotensin II-induced contraction. In addition, LEL oral administration resulted in the significant reduction in blood pressure of SHRs. Therefore, our study suggest that LEL may be an effective alternative for the treatment of hypertensive diseases. However, further researches on the active components and toxicity of LEL are needed.

Author Contributions: Conceptualization, S.S. and K.L.; methodology, S.S. and H.-Y.C.; software, S.S.; formal analysis, S.S. and Y.B.; investigation, S.S. and J.P.; resources, H.-Y.C. and K.L.; data curation, S.S.; writing—original draft preparation, S.S. and J.P.; writing—review and editing, S.S., Y.B. and K.L.; supervision, K.L. All authors have read and agreed to the published version of the manuscript.

Funding: This research received no external funding.

Institutional Review Board Statement: The animal study protocol was approved by the Institutional Animal Care and Use Committee of Kyung Hee University (approval number: KHSASP-23–506 on 17 November 2023).

Data Availability Statement: The original contributions presented in the study are included in the article; further inquiries can be directed to the corresponding author.

Conflicts of Interest: The authors declare no conflicts of interest.

References

1. Jagannathan, R.; Patel, S.A.; Ali, M.K.; Narayan, K.M.V. Global Updates on Cardiovascular Disease Mortality Trends and Attribution of Traditional Risk Factors. *Curr. Diabetes Rep.* **2019**, *19*, 44. [CrossRef]
2. Fuchs, F.D.; Whelton, P.K. High Blood Pressure and Cardiovascular Disease. *Hypertension* **2020**, *75*, 285–292. [CrossRef]
3. Niiranen, T.J.; Lyass, A.; Larson, M.G.; Hamburg, N.M.; Benjamin, E.J.; Mitchell, G.F.; Vasan, R.S. Prevalence, Correlates, and Prognosis of Healthy Vascular Aging in a Western Community-Dwelling Cohort: The Framingham Heart Study. *Hypertension* **2017**, *70*, 267–274. [CrossRef] [PubMed]
4. NCD Risk Factor Collaboration (NCD-RisC). Long-term and recent trends in hypertension awareness, treatment, and control in 12 high-income countries: An analysis of 123 nationally representative surveys. *Lancet* **2019**, *394*, 639–651. [CrossRef]
5. Oliveros, E.; Patel, H.; Kyung, S.; Fugar, S.; Goldberg, A.; Madan, N.; Williams, K.A. Hypertension in older adults: Assessment, management, and challenges. *Clin. Cardiol.* **2020**, *43*, 99–107. [CrossRef] [PubMed]
6. Muntner, P.; Hardy, S.T.; Fine, L.J.; Jaeger, B.C.; Wozniak, G.; Levitan, E.B.; Colantonio, L.D. Trends in Blood Pressure Control Among US Adults with Hypertension, 1999–2000 to 2017–2018. *JAMA* **2020**, *324*, 1190–1200. [CrossRef]
7. Alves-Silva, J.M.; Zuzarte, M.; Girão, H.; Salgueiro, L. Natural Products in Cardiovascular Diseases: The Potential of Plants from the Allioideae Subfamily (Ex-Alliaceae Family) and Their Sulphur-Containing Compounds. *Plants* **2022**, *11*, 1920. [CrossRef]
8. Rodríguez, L.; Mendez, D.; Montecino, H.; Carrasco, B.; Arevalo, B.; Palomo, I.; Fuentes, E. Role of *Phaseolus vulgaris* L. in the Prevention of Cardiovascular Diseases-Cardioprotective Potential of Bioactive Compounds. *Plants* **2022**, *11*, 186. [CrossRef]
9. Samtiya, M.; Aluko, R.E.; Dhewa, T.; Moreno-Rojas, J.M. Potential Health Benefits of Plant Food-Derived Bioactive Components: An Overview. *Foods* **2021**, *10*, 839. [CrossRef] [PubMed]
10. Souza, P.d.; Silva, R.d.C.V.d.; Mariano, L.N.B.; Dick, S.L.; Ventura, G.C.; Cechinel-Filho, V. Diuretic and Natriuretic Effects of Hesperidin, a Flavanone Glycoside, in Female and Male Hypertensive Rats. *Plants* **2023**, *12*, 25. [CrossRef] [PubMed]
11. Kamyab, R.; Namdar, H.; Torbati, M.; Ghojazadeh, M.; Araj-Khodaei, M.; Fazljou, S.M.B. Medicinal Plants in the Treatment of Hypertension: A Review. *Adv. Pharm. Bull.* **2021**, *11*, 601–617. [CrossRef]
12. Rastogi, S.; Pandey, M.M.; Rawat, A.K.S. Traditional herbs: A remedy for cardiovascular disorders. *Phytomedicine* **2016**, *23*, 1082–1089. [CrossRef]
13. Cao, Y.; Xuan, B.; Peng, B.; Li, C.; Chai, X.; Tu, P. The genus *Lindera*: A source of structurally diverse molecules having pharmacological significance. *Phytochem. Rev.* **2016**, *15*, 869–906. [CrossRef]
14. Ihm, S.-H.; Park, S.-H.; Lee, J.-O.; Kim, O.-R.; Park, E.-H.; Kim, K.-R.; Kim, J.-H.; Hwang, B.-H.; Youn, H.-J.; Oak, M.-H.; et al. A Standardized *Lindera obtusiloba* Extract Improves Endothelial Dysfunction and Attenuates Plaque Development in Hyperlipidemic ApoE-Knockout Mice. *Plants* **2021**, *10*, 2493. [CrossRef]
15. Shin, S.; Park, J.; Choi, H.-Y.; Lee, K. Hypotensive and Endothelium-Dependent Vasorelaxant Effects of Grayblue Spicebush Ethanol Extract in Rats. *Foods* **2023**, *12*, 4282. [CrossRef]
16. Lee, J.-O.; Oak, M.-H.; Jung, S.H.; Park, D.H.; Auger, C.; Kim, K.R.; Lee, S.-W.; Schini-Kerth, V.B. An ethanolic extract of *Lindera obtusiloba* stems causes NO-mediated endothelium-dependent relaxations in rat aortic rings and prevents angiotensin II-induced hypertension and endothelial dysfunction in rats. *N-S Arch. Pharmacol.* **2011**, *383*, 635–645. [CrossRef]
17. Ko, Y.-J.; Ahn, G.; Ham, Y.-M.; Song, S.-M.; Ko, E.-Y.; Cho, S.-H.; Yoon, W.-J.; Kim, K.-N. Anti-Inflammatory Effect and Mechanism of Action of *Lindera erythrocarpa* Essential Oil in Lipopolysaccharide-Stimulated Raw264.7 Cells. *Excli J.* **2017**, *16*, 1103–1113.
18. Yoon, C.-S.; Lee, H.; Liu, Z.; Lee, H.-K.; Lee, D.-S. Effects of Compounds Isolated from *Lindera erythrocarpa* on Anti-Inflammatory and Anti-Neuroinflammatory Action in BV2 Microglia and RAW264.7 Macrophage. *Int. J. Mol. Sci.* **2022**, *23*, 7122. [CrossRef]
19. Jung, J.; Shin, S.; Park, J.; Lee, K.; Choi, H.-Y. Hypotensive and Vasorelaxant Effects of Sanguisorbae Radix Ethanol Extract in Spontaneously Hypertensive and Sprague Dawley Rats. *Nutrients* **2023**, *15*, 4510. [CrossRef]
20. Shin, S.; Park, J.; Choi, H.-Y.; Bu, Y.; Lee, K. Vasorelaxant and Hypotensive Effects of *Galla chinensis* in Rats. *Int. J. Mol. Sci.* **2024**, *25*, 7962. [CrossRef]
21. Durand, M.J.; Gutterman, D.D. Diversity in Mechanisms of Endothelium-Dependent Vasodilation in Health and Disease. *Microcirculation* **2013**, *20*, 239–247. [CrossRef] [PubMed]
22. Chen, K.; Pittman, R.N.; Popel, A.S. Nitric oxide in the vasculature: Where does it come from and where does it go? A quantitative perspective. *Antioxid. Redox Sign* **2008**, *10*, 1185–1198. [CrossRef] [PubMed]
23. Kawabe, J.-I.; Ushikubi, F.; Hasebe, N. Prostacyclin in Vascular Diseases—Recent Insights and Future Perspectives. *Circ. J.* **2010**, *74*, 836–843. [CrossRef] [PubMed]

24. Cuíñas, A.; García-Morales, V.; Viña, D.; Gil-Longo, J.; Campos-Toimil, M. Activation of PKA and Epac proteins by cyclic AMP depletes intracellular calcium stores and reduces calcium availability for vasoconstriction. *Life Sci.* **2016**, *155*, 102–109. [CrossRef] [PubMed]
25. Touyz, R.M.; Alves-Lopes, R.; Rios, F.J.; Camargo, L.L.; Anagnostopoulou, A.; Arner, A.; Montezano, A.C. Vascular smooth muscle contraction in hypertension. *Cardiovasc. Res.* **2018**, *114*, 529–539. [CrossRef] [PubMed]
26. Hill-Eubanks, D.C.; Werner, M.E.; Heppner, T.J.; Nelson, M.T. Calcium Signaling in Smooth Muscle. *Cold Spring Harb. Perspect. Biol.* **2011**, *3*, a004549. [CrossRef] [PubMed]
27. Lee, C.-H.; Poburko, D.; Sahota, P.; Sandhu, J.; Ruehlmann, D.O.; Breemen, C.V. The mechanism of phenylephrine-mediated $[Ca^{2+}]_i$ oscillations underlying tonic contraction in the rabbit inferior vena cava. *J. Physiol.* **2001**, *534*, 641–650. [CrossRef]
28. Ghosh, D.; Syed, A.U.; Prada, M.P.; Nystoriak, M.A.; Santana, L.F.; Nieves-Cintrón, M.; Navedo, M.F. Calcium Channels in Vascular Smooth Muscle. *Adv. Pharmacol.* **2017**, *78*, 49–87.
29. Shah, K.; Seeley, S.; Schulz, C.; Fisher, J.; Rao, S.G. Calcium Channels in the Heart: Disease States and Drugs. *Cells* **2022**, *11*, 943. [CrossRef]
30. Jackson, W.F. Potassium Channels in Regulation of Vascular Smooth Muscle Contraction and Growth. *Adv. Pharmacol.* **2017**, *78*, 89–144.
31. Werner, M.E.; Ledoux, J. K^+ channels in biological processes: Vascular K^+ channels in the regulation of blood pressure. *J. Receptor. Ligand Channel Res.* **2014**, *7*, 51–60. [CrossRef]
32. Dogan, M.F.; Yildiz, O.; Arslan, S.O.; Ulusoy, K.G. Potassium channels in vascular smooth muscle: A pathophysiological and pharmacological perspective. *Fund. Clin. Pharmacol.* **2019**, *33*, 504–523. [CrossRef] [PubMed]
33. Cat, A.N.D.; Touyz, R.M. Cell Signaling of Angiotensin II on Vascular Tone: Novel Mechanisms. *Curr. Hypertens. Rep.* **2011**, *13*, 122–128.
34. Doris, P.A. Genetics of hypertension: An assessment of progress in the spontaneously hypertensive rat. *Physiol. Genom.* **2017**, *49*, 601–617. [CrossRef] [PubMed]
35. Doggrell, S.A.; Brown, L. Rat models of hypertension, cardiac hypertrophy and failure. *Cardiovasc. Res.* **1998**, *39*, 89–105. [CrossRef] [PubMed]
36. Tang, F.; Yan, H.-L.; Wang, L.-X.; Xu, J.-F.; Peng, C.; Ao, H.; Tan, Y.-Z. Review of Natural Resources with Vasodilation: Traditional Medicinal Plants, Natural Products, and Their Mechanism and Clinical Efficacy. *Front. Pharmacol.* **2021**, *12*, 627458. [CrossRef]
37. Rameshrad, M.; Babaei, H.; Azarmi, Y.; Fouladi, D.F. Rat aorta as a pharmacological tool for in vitro and in vivo studies. *Life Sci.* **2016**, *145*, 190–204. [CrossRef]
38. Rizzoni, D.; Agabiti-Rosei, E. Structural abnormalities of small resistance arteries in essential hypertension. *Intern. Emerg. Med.* **2012**, *7*, 205–212. [CrossRef]
39. Odukoya, J.O.; Odukoya, J.O.; Mmutlane, E.M.; Ndinteh, D.T. Ethnopharmacological Study of Medicinal Plants Used for the Treatment of Cardiovascular Diseases and Their Associated Risk Factors in sub-Saharan Africa. *Plants* **2022**, *11*, 1387. [CrossRef]
40. Uy, N.P.; Kim, J.H.; Kim, D.Y.; Ku, J.; Lee, S. Analysis of Marker Compounds in *Lindera erythrocarpa* from Diverse Geographical Regions of Korea. *Separations* **2024**, *11*, 252. [CrossRef]

nutrients

MDPI

Article

Botanical Bioflavonoid Composition from *Scutellaria baicalensis*- and *Acacia catechu*-Protected Mice against D-Galactose-Induced Immunosenescence, and Cyclophosphamide Induced Immune Suppression

Mesfin Yimam [1,*], Teresa Horm [2], Alexandria O'Neal [3], Paola Chua [4], Ping Jiao [1], Mei Hong [1] and Qi Jia [1]

1 Unigen Inc., 2121 South State Street, Suite #400, Tacoma, WA 98405, USA; pjiao@unigen.net (P.J.); meih@unigen.net (M.H.); qjia@unigen.net (Q.J.)
2 Department of Biology, Pacific Lutheran University, 12180 Park Ave. S, Tacoma, WA 98447, USA; teresamarie522@gmail.com
3 Seagen Pfizer, 21717 30th Dr SE, Bothell, WA 98021, USA; alexhoneal@gmail.com
4 Washington State Department of Health, 1610 NE 150th St, Shoreline, WA 98155, USA; chua.paolaa@gmail.com
* Correspondence: myimam@unigen.net

Abstract: Oxidative stress and chronic inflammation create a perpetual cycle in the elderly, where impaired immune function amplifies susceptibility to oxidative damage, and oxidative stress further weakens the immune response. This cycle is particularly detrimental to the respiratory system of the elderly, which is an easy target for constant exogenous harmful attacks during cold/flu season or under heavy air pollution. Herbal medicines that protect respiratory function are seen as safer alternatives to conventional therapies; however, there is limited availability of scientifically validated, safe, and effective natural supplements for these conditions. In this study, we evaluated a standardized bioflavonoid composition, UP446, that contains bioactives from the roots of *Scutellaria baicalensis* and the heartwoods of *Acacia catechu* as a natural and nutritional supplement for its antioxidative and immunoregulatory effects in oxidative stress-accelerated aging and chemically induced immune suppression mouse models. Immunosenescence was induced through the repeated subcutaneous inoculation of D-galactose (D-Gal) at a dose of 500 mg/kg/day in CD-1 mice. UP446 was administered orally at doses of 100 mg/kg and 200 mg/kg starting in the fifth week of immunosenescence induction. This study lasted a total of ten weeks. All mice received a quadrivalent influenza vaccine 2 weeks before termination. Whole blood, serum, spleen homogenate, and thymus tissues were processed for analysis. Cyclophosphamide (Cy)-induced immunosuppression was triggered by three consecutive injections of cyclophosphamide at 80 mg/kg/day, followed by the oral administration of UP446 for 18 days at doses of 100 mg/kg and 200 mg/kg. Blood was collected from each animal at necropsy, and serum was isolated for IgA and IgG ELISA analysis. UP446 was found to improve immune response, as evidenced by the stimulation of innate (NK cells) and adaptive immune responses (T cells and cytotoxic T cells), an increase in antioxidant capacity (glutathione peroxidase), the preservation of vital immune organs (the thymus), and a reduction in NFκB. UP446 also increased serum levels of IgA and IgG. The findings presented in this report demonstrate the antioxidative, anti-inflammatory, and immune-regulatory activities of UP446, suggesting its potential use in respiratory conditions involving immune stress due to aging, oxidative stress, and/or pathogenic challenges.

Keywords: immunosenescence; NK cells; T cells; antibody IgA; *Scutellaria baicalensis*; *Acacia catechu*; polyphenols; respiratory protection

1. Introduction

The pathophysiological association between pollution-induced oxidative stress and lung injury features a complex interplay with significant health implications. Environmental pollutants, such as PM2.5 particulate matter, can induce oxidative stress in the respiratory system [1]. This oxidative stress disrupts the balance between antioxidant defenses and reactive oxygen species (ROS) production, leading to cellular damage and inflammation in the respiratory system, especially the lungs. Oxidative stress is a key driver of inflammatory responses in lung tissues. It activates signaling pathways that promote the release of proinflammatory cytokines, chemokines, and damage-associated molecular patterns (DAMPs) like HMGB1, which collectively exacerbate inflammation and contribute to lung tissue injury [2].

HMGB1, in particular, is highlighted as a critical mediator in this process. It accumulates extracellularly in response to oxidative stress induced by pollutants, further amplifying inflammatory reactions and impairing immune cell functions. The buildup of HMGB1 in the airways and lungs is linked to a greater severity of inflammatory lung injury. The pathophysiology involves a cascade of events where oxidative stress initiates inflammatory responses, leading to tissue damage and compromising lung function. This relationship underscores the need for effective strategies to mitigate pollutant exposure, enhance antioxidant defenses, and potentially target HMGB1 to protect against pollution-induced oxidative stress and mitigate lung injury [3,4].

Previously, Yimam et al. (2023) proposed that reducing extracellular HMGB1 levels could restore immune cell functions and protect the lungs from oxidative stress-induced injuries. They tested their hypothesis using animal models and immune cell cultures exposed to oxidative stress or bacterial challenges [5]. UP446 was found to significantly reduce mortality rates, inhibit proinflammatory cytokines (TNF-α, IL-1β, IL-6) and chemokines (CINC-3), facilitate enhanced bacterial clearance from the lungs, and decrease airway protein levels, notably through the reduction in extracellular HMGB1 levels. Based on these facts, the authors concluded that the botanical composition is a potential intervention to protect the lungs against oxidative stress-induced injuries.

Oxidative stress, arising from an imbalance between antioxidants and reactive oxygen species (ROS), intensifies with age due to cumulative exposure to environmental factors, lifestyle choices, and declining cellular repair mechanisms. As such, the relationship among oxidative stress, old age, and compromised immunity has damaging consequences impacting overall respiratory health and susceptibility to diseases. In particular, the consequences are detrimental for the respiratory system as it is an easy target for constant exogenous harmful attacks during respiration [6].

In an aging population, physiological changes such as decreased antioxidant defenses and mitochondrial dysfunction contribute to heightened oxidative stress. This oxidative burden can impair immune function by disrupting signaling pathways crucial for immune cell activation, proliferation, and response to pathogens. Compromised immunity in aging is characterized by the reduced efficiency of innate and adaptive immune responses. This includes impaired phagocytosis by macrophages, the decreased production of cytokines and antibodies by lymphocytes, the dysregulation of inflammatory processes, and compromised immune responses [7,8]. These alterations make senior adults more vulnerable to infections due to chronic inflammatory conditions, less responsive to vaccination, and recover more slowly from illnesses. Moreover, oxidative stress-induced damage to immune cells and thymus tissues exacerbates age-related immune dysfunction. This can lead to a vicious cycle where impaired immunity further enhances susceptibility to oxidative stress and associated health challenges [9,10]. Therefore, addressing oxidative stress in aging populations through lifestyle interventions, the supplementation of dietary antioxidants, and potentially targeted interventions represents a promising approach to mitigate immune decline and improve overall health outcomes in senior adults.

Dietary supplements containing natural polyphenols offer a distinct advantage in oxidative stress management compared to basic antioxidant vitamins. These polyphenols, characterized by their diverse structures, potentially provide additional benefits beyond simple antioxidation [11]. Extracts of *Scutellaria baicalensis* roots and *Acacia catechu* heartwoods, along with their active bioflavonoid constituents present in the UP446 composition, are recognized for their notably varied antioxidant properties. For instance, baicalin, a flavonoid from the root of *S. baicalensis*, effectively scavenges DPPH free radicals (IC50 = 27.21 μM), inhibits CuSO4-induced lipid peroxidation (IC50 = 95.09 μM), demonstrates significant metal-chelating activity (IC50 = 352.04 μM) [12], and mitigates ROS production and MDA levels, while restoring SOD activity [13]. Similarly, catechins from green teas and the heartwoods of *Acacia catechu* demonstrate potent abilities to neutralize reactive oxygen and nitrogen species, effectively protecting against oxidative stress-induced lipid peroxidation and associated damage. They act as scavengers of reactive oxygen species (ROS) and chelators of metal ions. Additionally, catechins exert indirect antioxidant effects by inducing antioxidant enzymes, inhibiting pro-oxidant enzymes, and stimulating the production of phase II detoxification and antioxidant enzymes [14].

Hence, in the current study, we hypothesized that a standardized bioflavonoid composition, UP446, could mitigate oxidative stress and aging-associated declines in immune response. We proceeded to test this hypothesis using oxidative stress-accelerated immune senescence and chemically induced immune suppression models. Its antioxidation potential was also tested in vitro.

2. Materials and Methods

2.1. Composition

UP446 is a formulation containing extracts from heartwoods of *Acacia catechu* (*Senegalia catechu*) and roots of *Scutellaria baicalensis*, with preparation details disclosed in a US patent [15]. The process for preparing the extracts and the quantification of their full composition using High-Performance Liquid Chromatography (HPLC) have been described by Yimam et al. [16]. UP446 is a greenish yellow to brown powder with a standardized bioflavonoid composition that contains not less than 60% baicalin from *Scutellaria* as its major component and not less than 10% catechins from *Acacia* plus other minor bioflavonoids from both plants [16].

2.2. Animals

Mice (n = 130) (5 per cage) were housed in polypropylene cages and identified individually by tail numbers. Each cage was covered with a wire bar lid and filtered top (Allentown, NJ, USA). Cage cards were used to identify each cage, displaying the project number, test article, dose level, group, and animal numbers. Harlan T7087 soft cob bedding was used and changed at least twice a week. Animals were provided with fresh water and rodent chow diet #T2018 (Harlan Teklad, 370W, Kent, WA, USA) ad libitum, and housed in a temperature-controlled room (21.7–22.2 °C) on a 12 h light–dark shifts. In vivo experiments were carried out in accordance with institutional guidelines, consistent with the Guide for the Care and Use of Laboratory Animals with IACUC #s IAS-AO-030321 and IAS-PC-013123.

2.3. Antioxidant Assay by Oxygen Radical Absorbance Capacity (ORAC)

A UP446 sample was diluted in PBS (phosphate-buffered saline) to generate 500, 250, and 50 μg/mL solutions for testing. Two independent dilution series were prepared. A Trolox standard curve was generated to obtain 100, 50, 25, 12.5, and 6.125 μM in PBS. In total, 150 μL of fluorescein dilution was added to each well of a black 96-well plate, and 25 μL of Trolox dilutions or sample dilutions were added to triplicate wells. The plate was incubated at 37 °C for 10 min. AAPH (2,2′-Azodiisobutyramidine dihydrochloride) solution was prepared fresh for the assay using the assay buffer. The assay was initiated by adding 25 μL of the AAPH solution. The plate was inserted into the plate reader and a kinetic analysis of fluorescence decay was monitored every minute for 30 min at 37 °C. Trolox antioxidant activity was used as a standard to compare the test sample dilutions. The area under the curve of normalized decay curves was determined for each concentration of control and sample. The Trolox net AUC (Area Under the Curve) was used as a standard curve to calculate the Trolox equivalence of the test samples. Assay Plates: black 96-well clear bottom plates; reagents: phosphate-buffered saline (Lot: PBS104, ZenBio, Durham, NC, USA); assay buffer fluorescein (Lot: 041019, ZenBio); Trolox (Lot: 010622, ZenBio); AAPH (Lot: 0554100, ZenBio); instruments: Tecan Infinite F500 Plate Reader (Tecan, Männedorf, Switzerland)

2.4. Cyclophosphamide-Induced Immunosuppression in Mice

Purpose-bred male CD-1 mice (n = 50) were purchased from Charles River laboratories (Wilmington, MA, USA) at 22–24 g in body weight and acclimated for 1 week. Following acclimation, the animals were weighed for their baseline weights and randomized into 5 groups. There were 10 animals per group. The groups included G1 = control animals without cyclophosphamide, G2 = control model with cyclophosphamide, G3 = cyclophosphamide + levamisole 10 mg/kg, G4 = cyclophosphamide + UP446 100 mg/kg, and G5 = cyclophosphamide + UP446 200 mg/kg. Dosages were adjusted weekly based on bodyweight. Immunosuppression was induced by administering cyclophosphamide (Cy) at 80 mg/kg i.p. for 3 consecutive days. This study lasted for 3 weeks. For days 1–3, cyclophosphamide (Cy) was administered to all groups except the normal control group (−). Cy dissolved in saline was injected intraperitoneally at a 0.2 mL volume per animal. For days 4–21, mice were gavaged orally once per day for the indicated test materials. During the intervention period, the mice received no Cy. Animals were weighed weekly to determine subsequent dosages. Solutions were prepared for treatment groups in 0.5% CMC (Carboxy Methylcellulose) for oral delivery; 0.4 mL was administered per animal orally. On day 22 (Necropsy Day), blood was collected using a serum separator tube and was kept for at least 30 min before spinning at 11,000 rpm for 5 min at 4 °C. The serum was aspirated into microcentrifuge tubes (with about 400 μL yield) and stored in freezer until use.

UP446 was historically evaluated in our lab for multiple indications at 50, 100, 150, 200, and 250 mg/kg. Considering the repeated administration nature of the design, we selected 100 and 200 mg/kg for this study. For cyclophosphamide and levamisole dosages, we referenced previous reports [17]. Per protocol, the mice were monitored for 30 min after each gavage and daily thereafter for behavioral changes, food and water consumption, physical activity, appearance, and discharges from the eyes and orifices.

2.5. IgA and IgG ELISA

ELISAs for serum IgA and IgG were carried out following the manufacturer's instructions. ELISA products Abcam ab157719 and Abcam ab157717 (Abcam, Cambridge, UK) were used for IgG and IgA, respectively. While 0, 12.5, 25, 50, 100, 200, and 400 ng/mL concentrations were used for IgA standards; 0, 3.91, 7.81, 15.6, 31.3, 62.5, 125, and 250 ng/mL concentrations were used for IgG. Briefly, 100 μL of each standard and samples were pipetted in duplicate into predesignated wells. The micro titer plate was incubated at room temperature for sixty (60 ± 2) minutes. In total 100 μL of 1× enzyme–antibody conjugate was washed and added to each well, and incubated at room temperature for thirty (30 ± 2) minutes. The wells were washed and blotted. In total, 100 μL of TMB Substrate Solution was pipetted into each well and incubated in the dark at room temperature for ten minutes. After ten minutes, 100 μL of Stop Solution was added to each well, and the absorbance (450 nm) of the contents of each well was determined.

2.6. D-Galactose-Induced Accelerated Immune Senescence Model

Twelve-week-old purpose-bred male CD-1 mice (n = 80) were obtained from Charles River Laboratories, Inc. (Wilmington, MA, USA), and employed for the study post a one-week acclimation period. They were randomly divided into four groups of immunized and non-immunized groups. The groups were as follows: G1 = normal control + vehicle (0.5% CMC), G2 = D-galactose + vehicle, G3 = D-galactose + UP446 100 mg/kg, and

G4 = D-galactose + UP446 200 mg/kg. Each group consisted of 10 mice. Dosages were adjusted weekly based on bodyweight.

To induce accelerated immune senescence, mice were subcutaneously injected with D-galactose at a dosage of 500 mg/kg daily for 10 weeks. Treatment began four weeks after the induction started, at the beginning of week 5, with two doses of UP446 (100 mg/kg for the low dose and 200 mg/kg for the high dose), administered orally in a 0.5% CMC suspension for both the immunized and non-immunized groups. In week 8, all mice except those in the non-immunized groups received an intramuscular injection of 3 μg of the Fluarix quadrivalent influenza seasonal vaccine (2020–2021) (Lot # UJ477AA, 2020–2021) from GSK. This vaccine contained 60 μg of hemagglutinin per 0.5 mL single human dose, formulated with 15 μg of each of the four influenza strains: H1N1, H3N2, B-Victoria lineage, and B-Yamagata lineage.

Per the protocol, the mice were monitored for 30 min after each gavage and daily thereafter for behavioral changes, food and water consumption, physical activity, appearance, and discharges from the eyes and orifices.

The daily oral gavaging of UP446 was performed for six weeks, from the fifth week to the tenth week. At the time of necropsy, 14 days after immunization, 1 mL of blood was collected. A 110 μL aliquot was taken for a flow cytometry immunity panel in BD Microtainer® Tubes with Dipotassium EDTA (Lavender; BD, Franklin Lakes, NJ, USA). Serum was separated from the rest of the blood using SST and centrifuged at 1500 rpm for 10 min at 4 °C, yielding approximately 400 μL for antibody ELISAs and enzymatic assays. The thymus weights were recorded for every animal to determine thymus indices. The spleens were preserved on dry ice at necropsy and then transferred to −80 °C for future use.

2.7. Flow Cytometry Method

Whole blood was collected via cardiac puncture and transferred to EDTA blood collection tubes. Non-immunized samples were refrigerated overnight, while immunized samples were kept at room temperature on a nutator for up to 6 h. The samples were then transported on ice to the Flow Contract Site Lab (Bothell, WA, USA) for a 10-marker flow cytometry analysis. Doublets and debris were excluded, and the total cell population was identified using forward and side scatter gating. Fluorescent antibodies were used to distinguish cell populations. The blood was incubated for 15–20 min with the following antibodies: Mouse (m)CD45 V510 clone 30-F11 (BioLegend, San Diego, CA, USA, #103137), mCD3 APCCy7 clone 17A2 (BioLegend, #100221), mCD4 PECy7 clone GK1.5 (BioLegend, #100421), mCD8 AF700 clone 53-6.7 (BioLegend, #100729), mCD49b FITC clone DX5 (BioLegend, #108905), mLy6G APC clone 1A8 (BioLegend, #127613), mCD45R/B220 V605 clone RA3-6B2 (BioLegend, #103243), mNKp46 V421 clone 29A1.4 (BioLegend, #137611), mTCRγδ PE clone GL3 (BioLegend, #118107), and 7-AAD (BD or BioLegend, #420403). Red blood cells were lysed using PharmLyse (BD, #555899), and the samples were then centrifuged and resuspended in calcium- and magnesium-free DPBS (ThermoFisher Scientific, Waltham, MA, USA, #J67802K2) before being mixed with CountBright beads (ThermoFisher Scientific, #C36950). Flow cytometric data were acquired using a FACSCantoA, FACSCanto 10 Color flow cytometer (BD, Franklin Lakes, NJ, USA), and BD FACSDiva™ software version 9.0. Cell populations were determined by electronic gating based on the forward versus side scatter.

2.8. Serum Glutathione Peroxidase Activity

Mouse serum samples were tested for glutathione peroxidase activity using a Glutathione Peroxidase Assay Kit (Colorimetric) (Abcam ab102530) following the manufacturer's instructions. Briefly, a reaction mix was prepared by adding 33 μL of Assay Buffer, 3 μL of 40 mM NADPH solution, 2 μL of GR solution, and 2 μL of GSH solution. While standard wells were prepared at 100 μL standard dilutions; sample and reagent control wells were prepared at 50 μL per well. In total, 40 μL of Reaction Mix was added to the sample and reagent control wells only. The plate was incubated at room temperature for 15 min. The absorbance was read at OD 340 nm. In total, 10 μL of cumene hydroperoxide solution was added to the sample and reagent control wells only. The output (A1) was measured on a microplate reader at T1 at OD340 nm, and then incubated at 25 °C for 5 min, protected from light. The output (A2) was measured on a microplate reader at T2 at OD340 nm. Each sample was assayed in duplicate, and the absorbances of each sample were compared to a NADPH Standard curve.

2.9. Spleen Homogenate NFκB

Spleen tissues from the mice were homogenized in RIPA Lysis Buffer (50 mM Tris-HCl, pH 7.6, 150 mM NaCl, 1% NP-40, 0.5% Sodium deoxycholate, 0.1% SDS) at a concentration of 100 mg of tissue per mL of buffer, with three 10 s cycles on ice. The homogenates were then incubated on ice for 30 min to facilitate tissue lysis, followed by centrifugation at 16,000 RCF for 10 min at 4 °C. The supernatants were collected into new microcentrifuge tubes and stored at −80 °C. Spleen homogenates were subjected to SDS-PAGE, and the expression of markers was analyzed using primary antibodies against NFκB (Abcam, ab140751) with a Goat anti-Rabbit IgG Alexa Fluor Plus 488 secondary antibody, and anti-β-actin (Life Technologies, Carlsbad, CA, USA, MA5-15739-D680).

2.10. Serum Advanced Glycation End Products (AGEs)

Mouse serum samples were tested for AGEs using the Advanced Glycation End Product (AGE) Assay Kit (Colorimetric Assay, Abcam ab273298) according to the manufacturer's instructions. Briefly, samples were diluted to a protein concentration of 1 mg/mL with AGE Assay Buffer. In total, 10 μL of the diluted samples was added to the wells of a white 96-well plate, and the volume was adjusted to 200 μL with AGE Assay Buffer. A 1 mg/mL AGEs Positive Control was prepared by adding 2 μL of 10 mg/mL AGE Positive Control to 18 μL of AGE Assay Buffer. The same volume of the 1 mg/mL AGE Positive Control was added to the wells designated as "Positive Control", and the volume was adjusted to 200 μL with AGE Assay Buffer. The plate was incubated at room temperature for 5 min, protected from light. Fluorescence was measured at room temperature in end-point mode using a Tecan fluorescence microplate reader with excitation/emission settings of 360/460 nm.

2.11. Statistical Analysis

All descriptive data analyses were carried out using SigmaPlot 14.5 DA software (Palo Alto, CA, USA). The results are presented as the mean ± SD. Statistical significance among groups was assessed using single-factor analysis of variance and Student's *t*-test. *p*-values of 0.05 or less ($p \leq 0.05$) were regarded as statistically significant. Percent changes from the vehicle were determined using the following formula: % change = {(Mean value of Vehicle − Mean value of active test article)/Mean value of Vehicle} × 100. Flow cytometry data are reported as a percentage of all live white blood cells (CD45+ cells).

3. Results

3.1. Antioxidation Activity of UP446 as Measured by ORAC

UP446 has been found to possess strong antioxidation activity as measured in ORAC with a total ORAC value of 70,930 (μmole TE) per gram (Table 1). The ability of UP446 to neutralize Peroxyl Radicals, Hydroxyl Radicals, Peroxy Nitrite, Super Oxide Anion, and Singlet Oxygen radicals was measured and found as described in Table 1.

Table 1. Oxygen radical absorbance capacity of UP446.

Material	Specification	Peroxyl Radicals	Hydroxyl Radicals	Peroxy Nitrite	Super Oxide Anion	Singlet Oxygen	ORAC 5.0 (Total Score)
UP446	≥60% baicalin ≥10% catechins	8375	55,660	1397	4767	731	70,930

The ORAC result is expressed as the micromole Trolox equivalency (μmole TE) per gram. The ORAC (Trolox equivalents, TE) value was calculated by dividing the area under the sample curve by the area under the Trolox curve, with both areas being corrected by subtracting the area under the blank curve. Trolox was used as a positive control.

3.2. Immunomodulation Effect of UP446 on Cyclophosphamide-Induced Immunosuppression

All mice survived the duration of the study with no apparent changes suggestive of toxicity.

The injection of Cy to mice resulted in 4.38- and 2.03-fold significant reductions in the serum levels of IgA and IgG in CD-1 mice, respectively (Figures 1 and 2). These reductions were restored by the oral supplementation of UP446. In the case of IgA, mice administered with UP446 at 100 mg/kg and 200 mg/kg exhibited 3.26- and 3.06-fold increases in the serum IgA levels of mice, respectively (Figure 1). These increases in the level of serum IgA were statistically significant compared to the immune-suppressed group. In comparison to the controls, normal control and levamisole mice treated with the lower dosages (100 mg/kg UP446) showed no statistical significance difference, while the changes for the high dose (200 mg/kg) were significantly lower, $p = 0.02$.

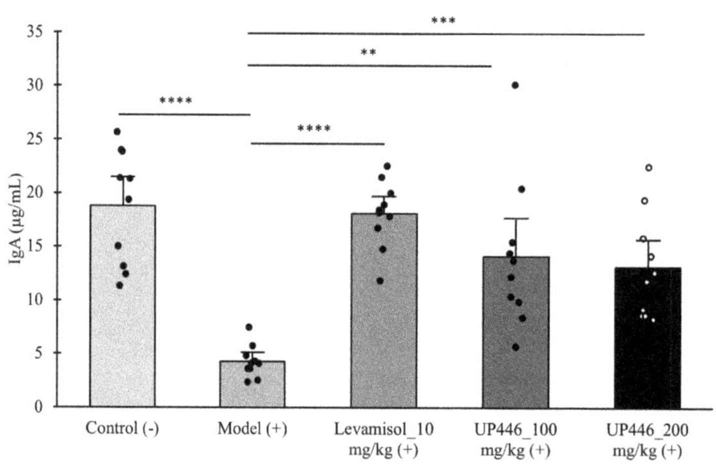

Figure 1. Immunomodulation effect of UP446 on cyclophosphamide-induced immunosuppression. Immunosuppression was induced by administering cyclophosphamide (Cy) at 80 mg/kg intraperitoneal for 3 subsequent days to CD-1 mice. Male CD-1 mice (n = 10) were treated with Levamisol_at 10 mg/kg, and UP446 at 100 and 200 mg/kg starting from day 4 for 18 days. The study lasted for 3 weeks. The control (−) group without cyclophosphamide (Cy) and model (+) received the vehicle 0.5% CMC (Carboxy Methylcellulose). The serum was separated at necropsy, and ELISA was carried out for IgA following the manufacturer's instructions. Data are expressed as the mean ± SD. ** $p \leq 0.01$ vs. model (+); *** $p \leq 0.001$ vs. model (+); **** $p \leq 0.0001$ vs. model (+). (+) represents model induction.

A similar immune modulation was observed for IgG. Animals administered with UP446 at 100 and 200 mg/kg showed 1.3- and 1.66-fold increases in the level of serum IgG, respectively. The induction in IgG was statistically significant for the 200 mg/kg of UP446 (Figure 2). The reference compound (levamisole) produced statistically significant 4.22- and 2.13-fold increases in the level of serum IgA and IgG, respectively. Both the 100 and 200 mg/kg UP446-treated groups showed no significant difference against levamisole; however, in comparison to the normal control, the low-dose group showed a statistically significant lower efficacy with no difference in efficacy to that of the high dose UP446.

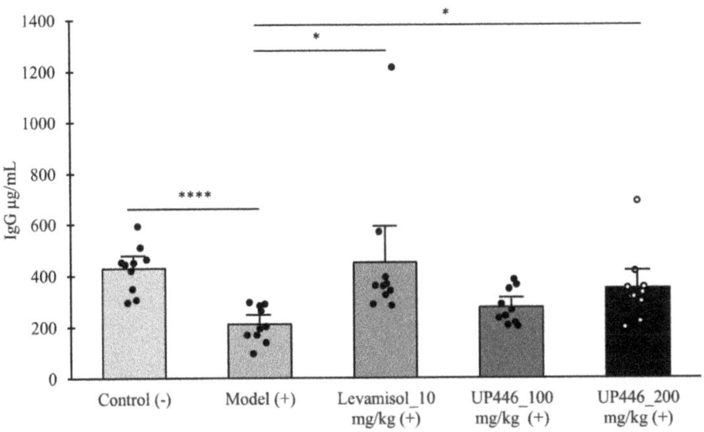

Figure 2. Immunomodulation effect of UP446 on cyclophosphamide-induced immunosuppression. Immunosuppression was induced by administering cyclophosphamide (Cy) at 80 mg/kg intraperitoneal for 3 subsequent days to CD-1 mice. Male CD-1 mice (n = 10) were treated with Levamisol_at 10 mg/kg, and UP446 at 100 and 200 mg/kg starting from day 4 for 18 days. The study lasted for 3 weeks. The control (−) group without Cy and model (+) received the vehicle 0.5% CMC (Carboxy Methylcellulose). The serum was separated at necropsy, and ELISA was carried out for IgG following the manufacturer's instructions. Data are expressed as the mean ± SD. * $p < 0.05$ vs. model (+); **** $p \leq 0.0001$ vs. model (+). (+) represents model induction.

3.3. *Effect of UP446 on the Immune Organ: The Thymus*

All mice survived the duration of the study with no apparent changes suggestive of toxicity.

In the immunized mice, D-Gal-induced immune senescence mice administered the vehicle displayed a significant 30.3% reduction in the thymus index compared to the normal control mice (Figure 3). This reduction was reversed by UP446 at both dosages. Mice treated orally with UP446 at 100 mg/kg and 200 mg/kg showed a 47.4% and 49.4% increase in the thymus index, respectively, compared to the vehicle-treated immune-compromised group (Figure 3). This reversal was statistically significant for both doses of UP446. These observations were comparable to the normal control, as there was no statistical difference between the normal control and UP446-treated mice for both the dosages.

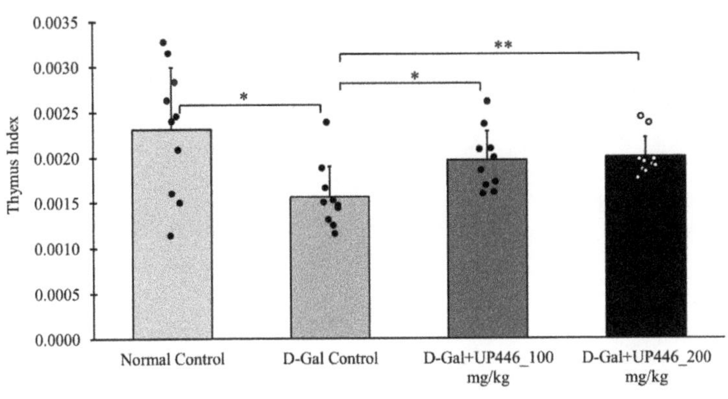

Figure 3. Impact of UP446 on the immune organ in immunized mice. Male CD-1 mice (n = 10) were inoculated subcutaneously with D-galactose at a dose of 500 mg/kg daily for 10 weeks to induce

accelerated aging. Starting in week 5, mice were treated orally with UP446 at doses of 100 and 200 mg/kg. They were immunized at the end of week 8 (beginning of week 9), and necropsy was performed at the end of week 10 (14 days post immunization). The normal control group, which did not receive D-galactose, and the D-galactose control group were both administered the vehicle, 0.5% CMC (Carboxy Methylcellulose). Thymus weights were measured for each animal to calculate thymus indices. Data are expressed as the mean ± SD * $p \leq 0.05$ vs. D-gal control; ** $p \leq 0.01$ vs. D-gal control. D-Gal: D-galactose.

Likewise, in non-immunized mice, UP446 at doses of 200 mg/kg and 100 mg/kg resulted in statistically significant increases in the thymus index, with increases of 27.4% and 31.6%, respectively, compared to the vehicle-treated immune-compromised mice (Figure 4). These observations were comparable to the normal control, as there was no statistical difference between the normal control and UP446-treated mice for both
the dosages.

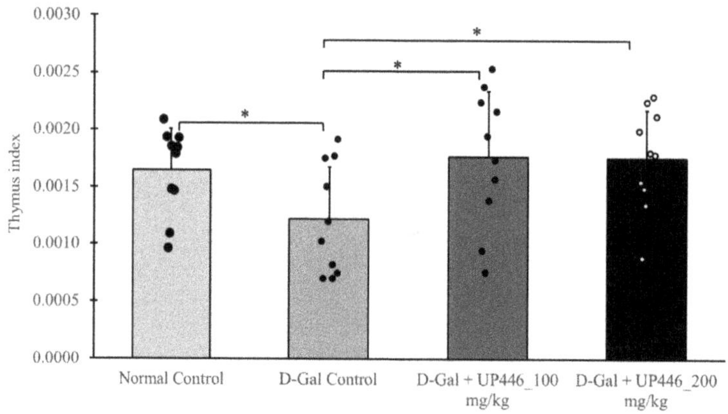

Figure 4. Impact of UP446 on the immune organ in non-immunized mice. Male CD-1 mice (n = 10) were inoculated subcutaneously with D-galactose at a dose of 500 mg/kg daily for 10 weeks to induce rapid aging. Starting in week 5, the mice received oral treatment with UP446 at doses of 100 and 200 mg/kg. Necropsy was performed at the end of week 10. The normal control group, which did not receive D-galactose, and the D-galactose control group were administered the vehicle, 0.5% CMC (Carboxy Methylcellulose). Thymus weights were recorded for each animal to determine thymus indices. Data are expressed as the mean ± SD. * $p \leq 0.05$ vs. D-gal control. D-Gal: D-galactose.

3.4. *Impact of UP446 on Circulating Immune Cell Populations in Immunized Mice*

The levels of circulating immune cells in the immunized groups of mice were assessed at the end of the study. Conveyed as a percentage of entire WBCs (CD45+ cells), the dosage correlated with 22.5% and 42.5% increases in natural killer cells (NK-cells), as recorded for mice administered UP446 at 100 and 200 mg/kg, respectively. These elevations of circulating NK-cells were statistically significant when compared to the D-gal + vehicle group. Changes for other immune cells were minimal (Table 2).

Table 2. Effect of UP446 on circulating immune cell populations in immunized mice †.

Cell Type	Normal Control	D-Gal Control	UP446_ 100 mg/kg	UP446_ 200 mg/kg
Lymphocytes	98.1 ± 0.9	98.8 ± 0.9	98.4 ± 1.2	98.2 ± 1.6
T cells	13.3 ± 3.1	13.0 ± 2.5	13.4 ± 3.3	15.8 ± 3.4 *
Helper T cells	8.5 ± 1.9	8.3 ± 1.5	8.0 ± 2.5	9.6 ± 2.5

Table 2. *Cont.*

Cell Type	Normal Control	D-Gal Control	UP446_ 100 mg/kg	UP446_ 200 mg/kg
Cytotoxic T cells (% of CD45+ cells)	4.2 ± 1.4	4.0 ± 1.2	4.4 ± 1.4	5.5 ± 1.3 *
Natural killer cells	4.2 ± 0.8	3.4 ± 1.7	4.8 ± 1.1 *	3.7 ± 2.1
Granulocytes	17.9 ± 6.7	23.1 ± 5.1	20.7 ± 4.4	20.0 ± 4.8
B cells	56.3 ± 7.1	50.4 ± 4.4	53.2 ± 6.5	51.2 ± 5.5
Gamma delta T cells	0.35 ± 0.15	0.38 ± 0.14	0.62 ± 0.81	0.33 ± 0.17
CD4+ Gamma delta T cells	0.15 ± 0.08	0.12 ± 0.08	1.00 ± 2.40	0.24 ± 0.20
CD8+ Gamma delta T cells	0.14 ± 0.12	0.12 ± 0.10	0.17 ± 0.18	0.13 ± 0.07

† values are expressed as % of total live cells; * $p \leq 0.05$.

3.5. Impact of UP446 on Circulating Immune Cell Populations in Non-Immunized Mice

Compared to the D-gal non-immunized group, the non-immunized group receiving 200 mg/kg of UP446 + D-gal showed a statistically significant 21.5% increase in T cell levels (CD3+ cells), conveyed as a percentage of total WBCs (CD45+ cells) (Table 3). A similar increase of 37.5% was also observed in CD3+CD8+ cytotoxic T cells in non-immunized D-gal mice treated with 200 mg/kg of UP446 (Table 3) At the lower dosage of 100 mg/kg, non-immunized D-gal mice administered UP446 exhibited a statistically significant 41.2% increase in natural killer cells (Table 3). Statistically non-significant moderate to minimal changes were observed for other immune cells at both dosages.

Table 3. Effect of UP446 on circulating immune cell populations in non-immunized mice †.

Cell Type	Normal Control	D-Gal Control	UP446_ 100 mg/kg	UP446_ 200 mg/kg
Lymphocytes	93.5 ± 2.7	97.0 ± 1.9	96.8 ± 1.7	96.1 ± 2.7
T cells	12.9 ± 1.9	10.6 ± 2.6	11.4 ± 2.6	10.1 ± 3.7
Helper T cells	8.9 ± 1.4	6.7 ± 1.8	7.5 ± 1.8	6.4 ± 2.0
Cytotoxic T cells	3.2 ± 1.0	3.2 ± 0.9	3.3 ± 0.9	3.1 ± 1.7
Natural killer cells	4.9 ± 2.0	4.0 ± 1.8	4.9 ± 1.6 *	5.7 ± 1.2 *
Granulocytes	20.0 ± 3.3	23.1 ± 5.2	24.2 ± 11.1	21.6 ± 7.4
B cells	51.0 ± 3.7	51.9 ± 6.3	48.9 ± 10.1	51.7 ± 8.9
Gamma delta T cells	0.65 ± 0.83	0.35 ± 0.14	0.29 ± 0.11	0.33 ± 0.08
CD4+ Gamma delta T cells	2.08 ± 5.98	0.25 ± 0.20	0.13 ± 0.09	0.22 ± 0.14
CD8+ Gamma delta T cells	0.11 ± 0.07	0.13 ± 0.08	0.07 ± 0.09	0.14 ± 0.11

† values are expressed as % of total live cells; * $p \leq 0.05$.

3.6. Impact of UP446 on a Transcription Factor NFκB

The SDS-PAGE assay showed that non-immunized D-gal mice treated with the vehicle had a 51.6% increase in the expression of NFκB. This elevation in the expression of the inflammatory transcription factor was mitigated by the use of UP446. A statistically significant 57.9% reduction in NFκB expression was observed in the non-immunized mice treated with 200 mg/kg of UP446 (Figure 5). When the reduction was compared to the normal control mice, it was not statistically significant.

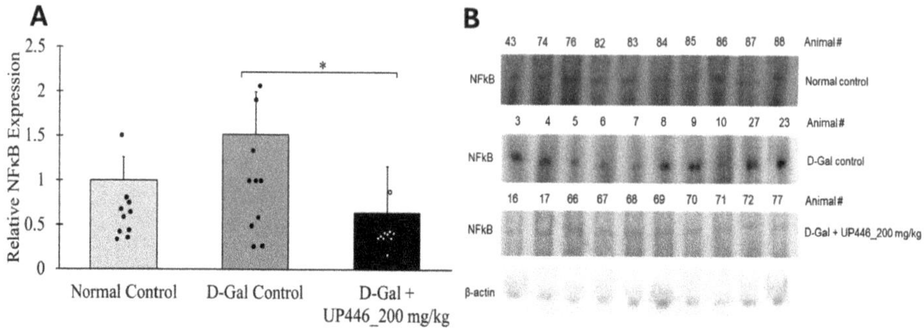

Figure 5. Effect of UP446 on a transcription factor NFκB on non-immunized mice. Male CD-1 mice (n = 10) were inoculated subcutaneously with D-galactose at a dose of 500 mg/kg daily for 10 weeks to induce rapid aging. Starting in week 5, the mice were treated orally with UP446 at a dose of 200 mg/kg. Necropsy was performed at the end of week 10. The normal control group, which did not receive D-galactose, and the D-galactose control group were administered the vehicle, 0.5% CMC (Carboxy Methylcellulose). During necropsy, spleens were placed on dry ice and subsequently stored at −80 °C for future use. Spleen homogenates were subjected to SDS-PAGE, and marker expressions were detected using primary antibodies against NFκB. (**A**) = Data are expressed as the mean ± SD. (**B**) = SDS-PAGE Gel. * $p \leq 0.05$ vs. D-gal control. D-Gal: D-galactose.

3.7. *Effect of UP446 on Advanced Glycation End Products (AGEs)*

Advanced glycation end products (AGEs) were assessed in serum samples from both non-immunized and immunized groups. The results indicate that the non-immunized D-Gal + UP446 groups had significantly lower serum AGEs compared to the non-immunized D-Gal mice treated with the vehicle. These reductions were dose-correlated, with 33.9% and 58.0% reductions in serum AGE levels for the 100 and 200 mg/kg UP446, respectively (Figure 6). When compared to the normal control, it was found that mice treated with the high dose (200 mg/kg UP446) showed statistically significant reductions.

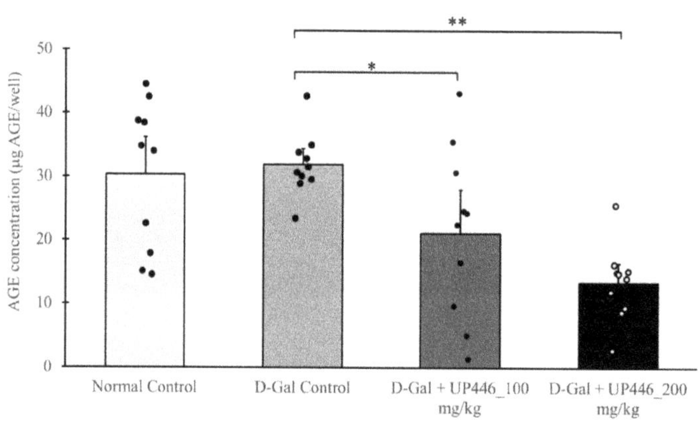

Figure 6. Effect of UP446 on advanced glycation end products (AGEs) on non-immunized mice. Male CD-1 mice (n = 10) received daily subcutaneous inoculation of D-galactose at 500 mg/kg for 10 weeks to induce rapid aging. Beginning in week 5, the mice were treated orally with UP446 at a dose of 200 mg/kg. Necropsy was performed at the end of week 10. The normal control group without D-gal and D-Gal control received the vehicle 0.5% CMC (Carboxy Methylcellulose). The serum was separated at necropsy and tested for AGEs using the Advanced Glycation End Products (AGEs) Assay Kit according to the manufacturer's instructions. Data are expressed as the mean ± SD. * $p \leq 0.05$ vs. D-gal control; ** $p \leq 0.01$ vs. D-gal control. D-Gal: D-galactose.

3.8. Effect of UP446 on Antioxidant Enzyme Glutathione Peroxidase In Vivo

Increased levels of antioxidant enzymes suggest that an intervention can improve the host's ability to counteract excess ROS. The activity of glutathione peroxidase (GSH-Px) was determined in serum samples from immunized mice. Dose-correlated, statistically significant increases of 20.1% and 23.3% in glutathione peroxidase activity were observed in immunized D-Gal mice treated with 100 and 200 mg/kg UP446, respectively (Figure 7). These changes were also statistically significant when they were compared against the normal control for both the dosages.

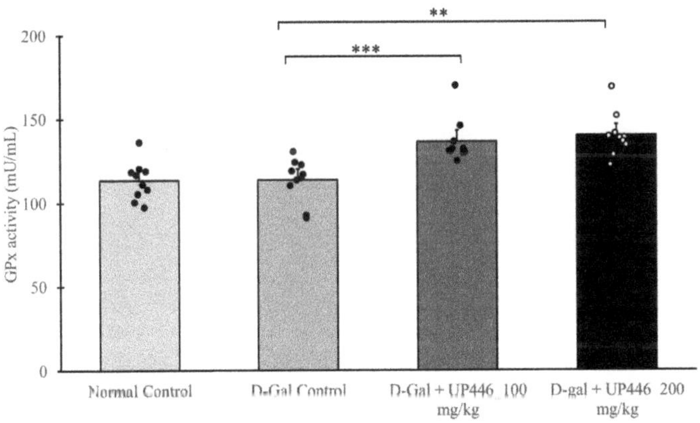

Figure 7. Antioxidation effect of UP446 on immunized mice. Male CD-1 mice (n = 10) received subcutaneous injections of D-galactose at a dose of 500 mg/kg daily for 10 weeks to promote accelerated aging. Starting in week 5, the mice were orally administered two doses of UP446 (100 or 200 mg/kg) and were immunized with 3 µg of the Fluarix quadrivalent vaccine at the end of week 8 (beginning of week 9). A necropsy was performed 2 weeks post immunization, at the conclusion of week 10. The serum was isolated at necropsy and tested for glutathione peroxidase activity using a Glutathione Peroxidase Assay Kit following the manufacturer's instructions. ** $p \leq 0.01$ vs. D-Gal control; *** $p \leq 0.001$ vs. D-Gal control.

4. Discussion

Immunosenescence, the gradual decline of the immune system associated with aging, is closely linked with oxidative stress. In the context of the respiratory system, oxidative stress exacerbates the decline in immune function by compromising the phagocytosis of immune cells and initiating chronic inflammation. The lungs are especially susceptible to oxidative stress due to constant exposure to environmental pollutants, pathogens, and other harmful agents inhaled during respiration. Immunosenescence further reduces the lungs' ability to respond to infections and repair damage, increasing vulnerability to respiratory diseases and chronic conditions. Together, oxidative stress and immunosenescence create a vicious cycle, where impaired immune function enhances susceptibility to oxidative damage, and oxidative stress further weakens the immune response. This highlights the importance of interventions to manage oxidative stress and support immune function in aging populations to protect lung health. Herbal medicines are seen as safer alternatives to conventional therapies for respiratory system support; however, most have not been scientifically validated for their safety and effectiveness as alternatives to natural supplements.

The data compiled in this report suggest that UP446 as a natural standardized bioflavonoid composition extracted from roots of *Scutellaria baicalensis* and heartwoods of *Acacia catechu* could potentially disrupt the oxidative stress and immunosenescence perpetual occurrence by mitigating age-associated immune decline and possessing strong antioxidation properties.

UP446 has shown strong antioxidation properties in vitro. The Oxygen Radical Absorbance Capacity (ORAC) measures a substance's ability to neutralize free radicals. Higher ORAC values suggest a greater capacity to neutralize free radicals. UP446 has been shown to possess high ORAC value at 70,930 (μmole TE) per gram. While the body typically maintains a balance between free radicals and antioxidants, excessive free radical production may require intervention. As such, UP446 could serve as a metabolism "sink" for the excess ROS to minimize their unwanted signaling and tissue damage.

Antioxidants such as UP446 play a crucial role in mitigating the formation and effects of advanced glycation end products (AGEs). By neutralizing reactive oxygen species and inhibiting glycation processes, UP446 helps reduce oxidative stress and AGE accumulation. In this study, age-associated increases in advanced glycation end products (AGEs) were observed in galactose-induced aging mice treated with a vehicle. UP446 significantly decreased the level of AGEs up to 58.0% after oral administration 200 mg/kg.

The accumulation of AGEs accelerates the decline in multiple system functions seen with aging, thus contributing to the aging process [18]. AGEs are known to cause extensive tissue damage by increasing inflammation and oxidative stress. Consistent with our findings, some antioxidants, like resveratrol, have shown potential in preventing AGE formation and breaking existing AGE cross-links, which can alleviate tissue damage and improve vascular health [19]. Therefore, incorporating UP446 into a daily supplement could promote wellness and combat age-related complications linked to AGE accumulation.

Glutathione peroxidase (GPx) is a key endogenous antioxidant enzyme that plays a critical role in protecting cells from oxidative stress [20]. It safeguards the body against oxidative stress-induced cellular dysfunction and contributes to overall health. Its regulation is significant in defending against age-related diseases. D-Gal induced aged mice supplemented with UP446 showed a dose-dependent increase in the level of GPx. Previously, individual components of UP446 have shown a significant increase in the levels of GPx. For example, the antioxidative actions of flavonoids quercetin and catechin were reported through the activation of hepatocyte glutathione peroxidase [21]. Similarly, multiple studies have shown the impact of baicalin in reversing the oxidative stress-induced reduction of glutathione peroxidase [22,23]. The results observed in our study could be the combined and synergistic effect of those two bioactive flavonoids in stimulating the production of GPx.

As maintaining adequate GPx function is crucial for supporting optimal antioxidant defense mechanisms and mitigating oxidative stress-related health risks, the inclusion of UP446 as a dietary supplement could provide significant benefits for overall health.

The NF-kB as a transcription factor complex is one of the cellular sensors that responds to oxidative stress and regulates gene expression [24]. Oxidative stress and the NF-κB signaling pathway are closely interconnected and significantly influence the aging process [25]. Reactive oxygen species (ROS) from oxidative stress activate NF-κB, a transcription factor that drives the gene expressions of many proinflammatory cytokines. This leads to chronic sterile inflammation, a key feature of aging and related chronic diseases. The feedback loop between ROS and NF-κB exacerbates oxidative damage and inflammation, contributing to immune cellular senescence and tissue function decline.

In the current study, aged D-gal mice treated with a vehicle showed a significant increase in the expression of NF-kB. In contrast, when these aged mice were orally administered UP446, the expression of NF-kB was significantly reduced. In agreement with our findings, it was previously reported that the inflammatory gene transcriptional factor controller, NF-κB, was down-regulated by UP446 in LPS-induced cellular models, highlighting the anti-inflammatory activities of UP446 [26]. Therefore, targeting oxidative stress and NF-κB activity through supplementation with UP446, which possesses antioxidant and anti-inflammatory properties, could promote healthy aging and mitigate age-related chronic diseases.

Repeated subcutaneous injections of D-galactose into mice induces significant oxidative stress that causes the damage of immune organ such as thymus, resembling alterations that take place during the normal aging process. A greater thymus index is associated with a more robust immune response [27]. The thymus indices for the normal control group and both UP446 + D-gal treatment groups were significantly greater than those of the vehicle + D-gal group, indicating that these treatments protect this immune organ from senescence induced by oxidative stress, which may result in enhanced production and maturation of immune cells. Supporting our findings with this model, Wei et al. reported that resveratrol promotes the proliferation of immune cells by improving thymus senescence and preventing involution [28].

Supplementation with the bioflavonoid composition UP446 induced mucosal immunity, in particular by increasing the production of IgA while also increasing IgG levels. This indicates the potential use of UP446 for lung protection and the preservation of mucosal immunity. A declined immune response, as reflected by reduced antibody production (IgA and IgG) and suppressed innate (NK cells) and adaptive immune cells (T cells and cytotoxic T cells), has been documented in the Endoxan-induced immune suppression and accelerated aging models. The reduced efficiency of both innate and adaptive immune responses, characterized by weakened macrophage activity, lower cytokine and antibody production, and impaired inflammatory regulation, are among the key features of immunosenescence. Supplementation with UP446 has reversed these age-associated and chemically induced immune senescence.

Specifically, the increase in IgA is crucial for the mucosal protection of the respiratory system, as this immunoglobulin is recognized for its ability to protect mucosal surfaces from microorganisms and foreign antigens. It also neutralizes bacterial products and helps eliminate pathogens or antigens that have penetrated the mucosal barrier [29]. These preclinical findings were later corroborated in a randomized, triple-blind, placebo-controlled clinical trial, where total IgA and IgG levels were found to be increased in senior participants who were orally supplemented with UP446 250 mg b.i.d compared to those on placebo. In the same clinical study, Lewis et al. reported that serum glutathione peroxidase (GSH-Px) was increased as a result of 500 mg/day UP446 supplementation, supporting the current preclinical antioxidation findings [30].

Herbal medicine is commonly used to support respiratory tract health during colds and flu. Among herbal remedies, echinacea, garlic, ginger, and elderberry have been used as complementary approaches to managing respiratory infections, with the potential to enhance immune function, reduce symptom severity, and shorten illness duration [31]. While some herbal treatments show notable promise, the scientific evidence varies, and their effectiveness may differ among individuals. In this regard, *Scutellaria baicalensis* has shown promise for treating the common cold, fever, and influenza. Research on cell cultures and mice has demonstrated that baicalin (the major active component of UP446) exhibits significant antiviral activity, particularly affecting virus budding in a dose-dependent manner. It functions as a neuraminidase inhibitor and is effective against various strains of influenza A virus both in vitro and in vivo [32]. The findings suggest that baicalin could be a valuable treatment option for influenza virus infections. In fact, a recent list of the top 30 herbs in Traditional Chinese Medicine (TCM) for treating respiratory infections ranked Radix *Scutellariae* as the second most utilized herb, with a 38% frequency in all TCM compositions for the treatment of respiratory tract infections [33]. We believe that the current findings depicted in this report will provide additional benefits in expanding the possible mechanisms of action of this botanical application, strengthening its traditional use for respiratory system support.

While the data depicted in this report are promising, this study and its interpretations are not without limitations. The thymus indices have not been confirmed with histopathology, leaving the question of immune organ protection by the supplement unresolved. Additionally, for NFkB analysis, the groups were run separately on SDS-PAGE, which casts doubt on the relative efficacy analysis data. Moreover, despite genetic and physiological similarities, mice and humans differ in immune system functioning and responses to pathogens. Although both species exhibit common aging signs, such as reduced immune function and increased susceptibility to diseases, the specific mechanisms and manifestations of aging can differ. These disparities can affect the accuracy of translating findings from mouse models to human conditions. Additionally, the controlled laboratory environment of mouse studies often does not account for the complex interactions and variability found in human populations, such as genetic diversity, environmental factors, and comorbid conditions. Consequently, while mouse models provide valuable insights, their results need to be carefully validated through human clinical trials before drawing definitive conclusions.

5. Conclusions

Collectively, supplementation with the standardized bioflavonoid composition of not less than 60% baicalin from the roots of *Scutellaria baicalensis* and not less than 10% catechin from the heartwoods of *Acacia catechu* has resulted in the protection of immune senescence from oxidative stress. In addition to the previously reported traditional usage, extracellular HMGB1 suppression activity and the increase in IgA from the human clinical trial, the data depicted in this report suggest that supplementation with UP446 could be beneficial for respiratory system support during immune-stressing conditions caused by aging, oxidative stress, and/or pathogen challenges.

Author Contributions: Conceptualization, M.Y., T.H. and Q.J.; data curation, M.Y., T.H. and Q.J.; formal analysis, M.Y., T.H. and Q.J.; funding acquisition, Q.J.; investigation, M.Y., T.H., A.O., P.C., P.J. and M.H.; methodology, M.Y., T.H., P.J. and M.H.; project administration, M.Y. and Q.J.; resources, Q.J.; supervision, M.Y. and Q.J.; validation, M.Y., T.H., P.J., M.H. and Q.J.; visualization, M.Y. and Q.J.; writing—original draft, M.Y.; writing—review and editing, M.Y. and Q.J. All authors have read and agreed to the published version of the manuscript.

Funding: No outside fund was acquired for this work. All expenses were covered by Unigen.

Institutional Review Board Statement: All animal experiments were conducted according to the institutional guidelines congruent with guidelines for the care and use of laboratory animals with IACUC #s IAS-AO-030321 and IAS-PC-013123 (approved on 3 March 2021 and 31 January 2023, respectively).

Informed Consent Statement: Not applicable.

Data Availability Statement: Data is contained within the article.

Acknowledgments: The authors would like to extend their utmost gratitude to Bill Lee, the owner of Econet/Unigen, Inc., who supported the fulfillment of this project.

Conflicts of Interest: M.Y., P.J., M.H. and Q.J. are current Unigen employees; therefore, they have competing financial interests.

References

1. Hou, T.; Zhu, L.; Wang, Y.; Peng, L. Oxidative stress is the pivot for PM2.5-induced lung injury. *Food Chem. Toxicol.* **2024**, *184*, 114362. [CrossRef] [PubMed]
2. Entezari, M.; Javdan, M.; Antoine, D.J.; Morrow, D.M.; Sitapara, R.A.; Patel, V.; Wang, M.; Sharma, L.; Gorasiya, S.; Zur, M.; et al. Inhibition of extracellular HMGB1 attenuates hyperoxia-induced inflammatory acute lung injury. *Redox Biol.* **2014**, *2*, 314–322. [CrossRef] [PubMed]
3. Patel, V.; Dial, K.; Wu, J.; Gauthier, A.G.; Wu, W.; Lin, M.; Espey, M.G.; Thomas, D.D.; Ashby, C.R., Jr.; Mantell, L.L. Dietary Antioxidants Significantly Attenuate Hyperoxia-Induced Acute Inflammatory Lung Injury by Enhancing Macrophage Function via Reducing the Accumulation of Airway HMGB1. *Int. J. Mol. Sci.* **2020**, *21*, 977. [CrossRef]
4. Wang, M.; Gauthier, A.; Daley, L.; Dial, K.; Wu, J.; Woo, J.; Lin, M.; Ashby, C.; Mantell, L.L. The Role of HMGB1, a Nuclear Damage-Associated Molecular Pattern Molecule, in the Pathogenesis of Lung Diseases. *Antioxid. Redox Signal.* **2019**, *31*, 954–993. [CrossRef] [PubMed]
5. Yimam, M.; Horm, T.; O'Neal, A.; Jiao, P.; Hong, M.; Brownell, L.; Jia, Q.; Lin, M.; Gauthier, A.; Wu, J.; et al. A Standardized Botanical Composition Mitigated Acute Inflammatory Lung Injury and Reduced Mortality through Extracellular HMGB1 Reduction. *Molecules* **2023**, *28*, 6560. [CrossRef]
6. Hajam, Y.A.; Rani, R.; Ganie, S.Y.; Sheikh, T.A.; Javaid, D.; Qadri, S.S.; Pramodh, S.; Alsulimani, A.; Alkhanani, M.F.; Harakeh, S.; et al. Oxidative Stress in Human Pathology and Aging: Molecular Mechanisms and Perspectives. *Cells* **2022**, *11*, 552. [CrossRef]

7. Guo, J.; Huang, X.; Dou, L.; Yan, M.; Shen, T.; Tang, W.; Li, J. Aging and aging-related diseases: From molecular mechanisms to interventions and treatments. *Signal Transduct. Target. Ther.* **2022**, *7*, 391. [CrossRef]
8. Teissier, T.; Boulanger, E.; Cox, L.S. Interconnections between Inflammageing and Immunosenescence during Ageing. *Cells* **2022**, *11*, 359. [CrossRef]
9. Luo, J.; Mills, K.; le Cessie, S.; Noordam, R.; van Heemst, D. Ageing, age-related diseases and oxidative stress: What to do next? *Ageing Res. Rev.* **2020**, *57*, 100982. [CrossRef]
10. Espino, J.; Pariente, J.A.; Rodríguez, A.B. Oxidative stress and immunosenescence: Therapeutic effects of melatonin. *Oxid. Med. Cell Longev.* **2012**, *2012*, 670294. [CrossRef]
11. Gao, Z.; Huang, K.; Yang, X.; Xu, H. Free radical scavenging and antioxidant activities of flavonoids extracted from the radix of *Scutellaria baicalensis* Georgi. *Biochim. Biophys. Acta (BBA) Gen. Subj.* **1999**, *1472*, 643–650. [CrossRef]
12. Paudel, K.R.; Kim, D.W. Microparticles-Mediated Vascular Inflammation and its Amelioration by Antioxidant Activity of Baicalin. *Antioxidants* **2020**, *9*, 890. [CrossRef]
13. Bai, X.; Yao, M.; Zhu, X.; Lian, Y.; Zhang, M. Baicalin suppresses interleukin-1β-induced apoptosis, inflammatory response, oxidative stress, and extracellular matrix degradation in human nucleus pulposus cells. *Immunopharmacol. Immunotoxicol.* **2023**, *45*, 433–442. [CrossRef]
14. Bernatoniene, J.; Kopustinskiene, D.M. The Role of Catechins in Cellular Responses to Oxidative Stress. *Molecules* **2018**, *23*, 965. [CrossRef] [PubMed]
15. Jia, Q. Formulation of a Mixture of Free-B-Ring Flavonoids and Flavans as a Therapeutic Agent. U.S. Patent US7514469B2, 7 April 2009.
16. Yimam, M.; Zhao, Y.; Ma, W.; Jia, Q.; Do, S.-G.; Shin, J.-H. 90-day oral toxicity study of UP446, a combination of defined extracts of *Scutellaria baicalensis* and *Acacia catechu*, in rats. *Food Chem. Toxicol.* **2010**, *48*, 1202–1209. [CrossRef] [PubMed]
17. Feng, H.; Fan, J.; Lin, L.; Liu, Y.; Chai, D.; Yang, J. Immunomodulatory Effects of Phosphorylated *Radix Cyathulae officinalis* Polysaccharides in Immunosuppressed Mice. *Molecules* **2019**, *24*, 4150. [CrossRef]
18. Semba, R.D.; Nicklett, E.J.; Ferrucci, L. Does accumulation of advanced glycation end products contribute to the aging phenotype? *J. Gerontol. A Biol. Sci. Med. Sci.* **2010**, *65*, 963–975. [CrossRef]
19. Maleki, V.; Foroumandi, E.; Hajizadeh-Sharafabad, F.; Kheirouri, S.; Alizadeh, M. The effect of resveratrol on advanced glycation end products in diabetes mellitus: A systematic review. *Arch. Physiol. Biochem.* **2022**, *128*, 253–260. [CrossRef]
20. Averill-Bates, D.A. The antioxidant glutathione. *Vitam. Horm.* **2023**, *121*, 109–141.
21. Nagata, H.; Takekoshi, S.; Takagi, T.; Honma, T.; Watanabe, K. Antioxidative action of flavonoids, quercetin and catechin, mediated by the activation of glutathione peroxidase. *Tokai J. Exp. Clin. Med.* **1999**, *24*, 1–11.
22. Ma, L.; Wu, F.; Shao, Q.; Chen, G.; Xu, L.; Lu, F. Baicalin Alleviates Oxidative Stress and Inflammation in Diabetic Nephropathy via Nrf2 and MAPK Signaling Pathway. *Drug Des. Dev. Ther.* **2021**, *15*, 3207–3221. [CrossRef] [PubMed]
23. Fang, J.; Wang, H.; Zhou, J.; Dai, W.; Zhu, Y.; Zhou, Y.; Wang, X.; Zhou, M. Baicalin provides neuroprotection in traumatic brain injury mice model through Akt/Nrf2 pathway. *Drug Des. Dev. Ther.* **2018**, *12*, 2497–2508. [CrossRef] [PubMed]
24. Helenius, M.; Hänninen, M.; Lehtinen, S.K.; Salminen, A. Aging-induced up-regulation of nuclear binding activities of oxidative stress responsive NF-kB transcription factor in mouse cardiac muscle. *J. Mol. Cell. Cardiol.* **1996**, *28*, 487–498. [CrossRef] [PubMed]
25. Galli, F.; Marcantonini, G.; Giustarini, D.; Albertini, M.C.; Migni, A.; Zatini, L.; Gioiello, A.; Rossi, R.; Bartolini, D. How Aging and Oxidative Stress Influence the Cytopathic and Inflammatory Effects of SARS-CoV-2 Infection: The Role of Cellular Glutathione and Cysteine Metabolism. *Antioxidants* **2022**, *11*, 1366. [CrossRef] [PubMed]
26. Tseng-Crank, J.; Sung, S.; Jia, Q.; Zhao, Y.; Burnett, B.; Park, D.R.; Woo, S.S. A medicinal plant extract of Scutellaria Baicalensis and *Acacia catechu* reduced LPS-stimulated gene expression in immune cells: A comprehensive genomic study using QPCR, ELISA, and microarray. *J. Diet. Suppl.* **2010**, *7*, 253–272. [CrossRef] [PubMed]
27. Thapa, P.; Farber, D.L. The Role of the Thymus in the Immune Response. *Thorac. Surg. Clin.* **2019**, *29*, 123–131. [CrossRef]
28. Wei, T.T.; Li, M.J.; Guo, L.; Xie, Y.D.; Chen, W.H.; Sun, Y.; Liu, G.H.; Ding, Y.; Chai, Y.R. Resveratrol ameliorates thymus senescence changes in D-galactose induced mice. *Microbiol. Immunol.* **2020**, *64*, 620–629. [CrossRef]
29. Pilette, C.; Ouadrhiri, Y.; Godding, V.; Vaerman, J.P.; Sibille, Y. Lung mucosal immunity: Immunoglobulin-A revisited. *Eur. Respir. J.* **2001**, *18*, 571–588. [CrossRef]
30. Lewis, E.D.; Crowley, D.C.; Guthrie, N.; Evans, M. Role of *Acacia catechu* and *Scutellaria baicalensis* in Enhancing Immune Function Following Influenza Vaccination of Healthy Adults: A Randomized, Triple-Blind, Placebo-Controlled Clinical Trial. *J. Am. Nutr. Assoc.* **2023**, *42*, 678–690. [CrossRef]
31. Mousa, H.A. Prevention and Treatment of Influenza, Influenza-Like Illness, and Common Cold by Herbal, Complementary, and Natural Therapies. *J. Evid. Based Complement. Altern. Med.* **2017**, *22*, 166–174. [CrossRef]
32. Ding, Y.; Dou, J.; Teng, Z.; Yu, J.; Wang, T.; Lu, N.; Wang, H.; Zhou, C. Antiviral activity of baicalin against influenza A (H1N1/H3N2) virus in cell culture and in mice and its inhibition of neuraminidase. *Arch. Virol.* **2014**, *159*, 3269–3278. [CrossRef] [PubMed]
33. Ge, H.; Wang, Y.F.; Xu, J.; Gu, Q.; Liu, H.B.; Xiao, P.G.; Zhou, J.; Liu, Y.; Yang, Z.; Su, H. Anti-influenza agents from Traditional Chinese Medicine. *Nat. Prod. Rep.* **2010**, *27*, 1758–1780. [CrossRef] [PubMed]

nutrients

MDPI

Article

Euglena gracilis Enhances Innate and Adaptive Immunity through Specific Expression of Dectin-1 in CP-Induced Immunosuppressed Mice

Hwan Hee Lee [1,2], Ji-Yeon Seong [2], Hyojeung Kang [3,*] and Hyosun Cho [1,2,*]

1 College of Pharmacy, Duksung Women's University, Seoul 01369, Republic of Korea; oeo3oeo@gmail.com
2 Duksung Innovative Drug Center, Duksung Women's University, Seoul 01369, Republic of Korea; sjyne@duksung.ac.kr
3 Vessel-Organ Interaction Research Center, VOICE (MRC), Cancer Research Institute, College of Pharmacy, Kyungpook National University, Daegu 41566, Republic of Korea
* Correspondence: hkang72@knu.ac.kr (H.K.); hyosun1102@duksung.ac.kr (H.C.); Tel.: +82-53-950-8569 (H.K.); +82-2-901-8678 (H.C.)

Abstract: Background: *Euglena gracilis* (*E. gracilis*), a species of unicellular algae, can accumulate large amounts of β-1,3-glucan paramylon, a polysaccharide, in its cytoplasm and has recently attracted interest as a bioproduct due to its various health benefits. In this study, the immune-enhancing effect of *E. gracilis* powder (EP) was investigated in vitro and in vivo. Methods: In vitro, the production of NO and cytokines and the mechanism of the signaling pathway of β-1,3-glucan were identified in RAW264.7 cells. In vivo, cyclophosphamide-induced (CP-induced) immunosuppressed C57BL/6 female mice were orally administered with three different concentrations (100, 300, and 600 mg/kg) of EP daily. After 14 days, the organs and whole blood were collected from each animal for further study. Results: The weight loss of CP-treated mice was reversed by treatment with EP to levels comparable to those of control mice. In addition, the frequencies of NK1.1$^+$, CD3$^+$, CD4$^+$, CD8$^+$, and B220$^+$ in immune cells isolated from the spleen were increased by EP treatment compared with water or RG. The secretion of TNF-α, IFN-γ, and IL-12 from splenocytes was also increased by EP treatment, as was the level of IgM in the serum of the mice. Finally, EP treatment specifically upregulated the expression of dectin-1 in the liver of CP-treated mice. Conclusions: *E. gracilis* could be a good candidate for a natural immune stimulator in the innate and adaptive response by secreting TNF-α, IFN-γ, and IL-12 through stimulating dectin-1 expression on the surface of immune cells.

Keywords: *E. gracilis*; β-1,3-glucan; immune-enhancing effect; immunosuppressed mice; dectin-1; cyclophosphamide

1. Introduction

The immune system consists of innate and adaptive immunity, and it plays a critical role in resisting pathogenic infection and in maintaining homeostasis. Innate immunity is the first line of defense against pathogens and includes phagocytes, which consist of neutrophils, dendritic cells, blood monocytes, and tissue macrophages. Phagocytes identify pathogens through pattern recognition receptors (PRRs), including Toll-like receptors (TLRs). This recognition can lead to the direct killing of pathogens or facilitate the activation of T cells, which are integral to the adaptive immune response, by presenting antigens [1]. Lymphocytes include natural killer (NK) cells, which are part of the innate immune system, and T cells and B cells, which are responsible for adaptive immune responses. NK cells are most abundant in the peripheral blood and are also present in other organs [2]. Their function is to directly kill virus-infected or transformed cells without prior sensitization [3], and they have recently been shown to produce several cytokines that help other immune cells [4]. In adaptive immunity, T or B lymphocytes can remember previous invaders and develop an intense response to a second invasion. Therefore, the coordination between different immune cells is very important to elicit an appropriate immune response to a foreign agent [5,6].

E. gracilis is a species of unicellular algae found in most freshwater biotopes and is characterized by being mixotrophic, capable of both prototrophic and heterotropic feeding [7,8]. Recent studies have highlighted the potential of bioproducts derived from *E. gracilis* due to its diverse range of components, including the main component β-1,3-glucan paramylon, as well as amino acids, provitamins, and lipids [9–11]. In particular, β-1,3-glucan paramylon is a reserve polysaccharide and can accumulate in large amounts (>80%) depending on the cultivation conditions of *E. gracilis* [8,12]. Other derived β-glucans (e.g., yeast, oat) are already known to have various bioactivities, including immunostimulatory and antimicrobial effects in animals and humans [13–15].

Dectin-1 is a C-type lectin receptor (CLR) that recognizes β-glucans from fungi, plants, and algae [16]. It is expressed mainly on myeloid cells but can also be found on some lymphocytes [17]. Binding of β-glucans to dectin-1 on myeloid cells results in the production of several cytokines and reactive oxygen species (ROS) involved in myeloid cell activation reactions [18,19]; however, this depends on the structural conformations of the β-glucans.

Cyclophosphamide (CP) is a drug used in chemotherapy to treat many cancers, including lymphoma, multiple myeloma, and breast cancer [20]. Its mechanism in cancer is to interfere with protein synthesis through DNA and RNA cross-linking, resulting in apoptosis of cancer cells and inhibition of cell cycle [21,22]. However, CP can reduce the number of lymphocytes such as T cells and B cells [21,22]. In this respect, it is often used as a potent immunosuppressive agent in animal experiments to investigate the immunomodulatory effects of certain substances in vivo [23,24].

Several studies have demonstrated the effect of *E. gracilis* on innate and adaptive immunity through in vitro and in vivo experiments, but the mechanism is still unclear. The immune system is critical to maintaining body homeostasis, so it must be controlled to ensure that immune responses do not become excessively elevated or depressed. CP is known to induce the depression of lymphocytes in mice, which disrupts the homeostasis of the immune system. In light of this, we investigated the immune-enhancing effect of EP containing large amounts of β-1,3-glucan paramylon using CP-induced immunosuppressed mice.

2. Materials and Methods

2.1. Specimen Preparation

β-1,3-glucan derived from *E. gracilis* was sourced from Sigma-Aldrich Inc. (St. Louis, MO, USA). For in vitro study, β-1,3-glucan was treated with 0.5 mol/L NaOH and stirred until a homogeneous solution was achieved. It was then precipitated using cold 98% ethanol and collected by centrifugation at 12,000× *g* for 10 min at 4 °C. The specimen was suspended in 40 mL of deionized water and subsequently diluted, following the method described in [13]. BioGlena^{TM}, EP containing over 50% β-1,3-glucan, was acquired from JUYEONG NS Co., Ltd. (Seoul, Republic of Korea), which is supplied by Algatechnologies Ltd. (Kibbutz Ketura, Israel). For the in vivo study, EP was dissolved in drinking water.

2.2. Cell Culture and Treatment

The mouse macrophage cell line RAW264.7 was obtained from the Korea Cell Line Bank (KCLB, Seoul, Republic of Korea). The cells were maintained in Dulbecco's modified Eagle's medium (DMEM, Gibco, Grand Island, NY, USA) supplemented with 10% fetal bovine serum (FBS, Gibco) and 1% penicillin and streptomycin (Gibco) at 37 °C in a humidified environment with 5% CO_2. For in vitro experiments, the cells were seeded into plates and incubated overnight (18–24 h) before being treated with β-1,3-glucan for 24 h. The supernatant was then collected for cytokine analysis, while the cell lysates were prepared for studying the underlying mechanism.

2.3. CCK-8 Assay

To assess the cytotoxicity of β-1,3-glucan on RAW264.7 cells, the cells were seeded into a 96-well flat-bottom plate and exposed to lipopolysaccharide (LPS) at 1 μg/mL or varying concentration of β-1,3-glucan (0, 50, 100, 250, 500, and 1000 μg/mL) for 24 h. Following this, the CCK-8 solution was added to each well, and the cells were incubated for an additional 3 h. The absorbance was then read at 490 nm using a microplate reader (BMG Labtech, Ortenberg, Germany).

2.4. Nitric Oxide (NO) Assay

Cell-free supernatants were collected from RAW264.7 cells that had been treated with LPS or varying concentrations of β-1,3-glucan (0, 50, 100, 250, and 500 μg/mL) for 24 h to assess the production of nitric oxide (NO) metabolites. The nitrite/nitrate assay kit (Sigma-Aldrich) was used following the protocol provided by the manufacturer. The absorbance was measured at 540 nm using a microplate reader.

2.5. Cytokine Analysis

Supernatants from RAW264.7 cells treated with LPS or various concentrations of β-1,3-glucan, as well as from mouse splenocytes incubated with or without concanvalin A (ConA, 10 μg/mL) for 72 h, were collected for cytokine analysis. Levels of TNF-α and IL-1β were measured using a mouse Uncoated ELISA kit (Invitrogen, Waltham, MA, USA), while IL-6, IL-12, and IFN-γ were quantified using a mouse ELISA kit (BD Biosciences, Franklin Lakes, NJ, USA). All procedures followed the protocols provided by the manufacturers. Absorbance readings were taken at 450 nm using a microplate reader (BMG Labtech).

2.6. Western Blot Analysis

RAW264.7 cells were exposed to LPS or different concentrations of β-1,3-glucan (50, 100, 250, and 500 μg/mL) for 24 h. After treatment, the cells were lysed using a protein extraction buffer (Intron, Seoul, Republic of Korea) containing phosphatase inhibitors. Protein concentration was determined using the Bradford (Coomassie blue) assay. Proteins were then separated by electrophoresis, transferred onto polyvinylidene fluoride (PVFD) microporous membrane with a 0.2 μm pore (Millipore, Burlington, MA, USA), and subjected to immunoblotting with primary and secondary antibodies. Protein bands were visualized using the Chemi-Doc imaging system (Millipore) and enhanced chemiluminescence detection solution. The primary antibodies used included anti-TLR6, anti-pERK (p42/p44), anti-pNF-κB (all from Cell Signaling, Danvers, MA, USA), anti-dectin-1 (Abcam, Cambridge, UK), and anti-β-actin (Sigma-Aldrich, St. Louis, MO, USA). The secondary antibodies, anti-mouse IgG and anti-rabbit IgG, were obtained from Cell Signaling Technology (CST) Inc. (Danvers, MA, USA).

2.7. In Vivo Experiments Using Immunosuppressed C57BL/6 Mice

All in vivo studies were conducted following the guidelines set by the National Research Council's Guide for Care and Use of Laboratory Animals. The study protocol received approval from the Animal Experiments Committee of Duksung Women's University (permit number: 2024-004-026). Female C57BL/6 mice, 5 weeks old, were obtained from JABIO Inc. (Seoul, Republic of Korea). Prior to the experiment, all mice were acclimated in the laboratory for one week under controlled conditions, including a temperature of 23 ± 2 °C and a 12-h light/dark cycle. The mice were randomly divided into six groups (n = 8 per group) and received intraperitoneal injections of 150 mg/kg of CP on days 1 and 3, except for the control group (NC) which received only drinking water. The groups were as follows: (1) control with drinking water (NC), (2) water with CP, (3) 10 mg/kg red ginseng (RG) with CP, (4) 100 mg/kg EP with CP, (5) 300 mg/kg EP with CP, and (6) 600 mg/kg EP with CP. Each test substance was administered orally once daily for 14 days. Throughout the study, mice were weighed daily, and at the end of the experiment, the weight of the liver, spleen, and thymus were recorded.

2.8. Complete Blood Cell Count (CBC) Analysis

After 14 days, the mice were euthanized, and whole blood samples were collected for complete blood count (CBC) analysis. The total white blood cell (WBC) count, as well as the percentages of neutrophil (NEU), lymphocyte (LYM), monocyte (MONO), eosinophil (EOS), and basophil (BASO), were measured. Additional parameters such as red blood cell (RBC) count, platelet count, hemoglobin concentration (HGB), mean corpuscular volume (MCV), mean corpuscular hemoglobin (MCH), and mean corpuscular hemoglobin concentration (MCHC) were also assessed. These measurements were performed using an automated hematology analyzer (XN-100, Sysmex, Kobe, Japan).

2.9. Antibodies (IgM, IgG) Analysis

For antibody analysis, serum was separated from the whole blood of mice, and splenocytes were isolated from their spleen. The levels of IgM and IgG antibodies were measured using a mouse Uncoated ELISA (Invitrogen). The absorbance was recorded at 450 nm using a microplate reader (BMG Labtech).

2.10. Splenocyte Proliferation Assay

Splenocyte proliferation in response to EP was assessed using Cell Counting Kit-8 (CCK-8, Dojindo, Japan). Briefly, splenocytes were seeded in a 96-well flat-bottom plate at a density of 1×10^5 cells per well, with or without concanavalin (ConA, 10 μg/mL), and incubated for 72 h. After incubation, CCK-8 solution was added to each well and allowed to incubate for another 3 h. The absorbance was measured at 450 nm using a microplate reader.

2.11. Cell Surface Antigens Analysis by Flow Cytometry

Spleen cells from mice were stained with a combination of mouse anti-NK1.1-APC and anti-CD3-PE, a combination of anti-CD4-PE and anti-CD8-APC, and anti-B220-PE antibodies (all from BD Biosciences, Franklin Lakes, NJ, USA) for 30 min in the dark. After staining, the cells were analyzed using flow cytometry (Novocyte Flow Cytometer, ACEA Biosciences, Santa Clara, CA, USA). The positive cell populations were identified by comparing the results with predefined cutoff values obtained from unstained control cells, as previously described [23].

2.12. Immunohistochemistry (IHC) Staining

Mouse liver tissues were fixed using the paraffin embedding technique. Prior to antibody staining and blotting, the paraffin was removed with xylene, followed by dehydration with ethanol and treatment with 3% hydrogen peroxide (H_2O_2) diluted in methanol. Subsequently, the tissues were incubated with the primary antibody (m-dectin-1), followed by the secondary antibody. The tissues were then treated with avidin/biotin and a DAB substrate. After staining with hematoxylin, the tissues were mounted. Protein expression in the tissues was examined using light microscopy at magnifications of 40× and 200×.

2.13. Statistics

To ensure the significance of results in vitro experiments, all assays were conducted in triplicate, and the data are presented as mean ± SD. Both in vitro and in vivo data were analyzed using GraphPad Prism version 5.03 for Windows (GraphPad Software, www.graphpad.com (accessed on 15 September 2024)). Mean comparisons were performed using *t*-tests or one-way ANOVA followed by Tukey's multiple comparison test. A *p*-value of less than 0.05 was considered statistically significant.

3. Results

3.1. Production of Nitric Oxide (NO) in RAW264.7 Cells by β-1,3-Glucan

The production of NO metabolites by macrophage in response to β-1,3-glucan was investigated in RAW264.7 cells using a nitrite/nitrate assay kit. We first identified the cell cytotoxicity to β-1,3-glucan using the CCK-8 assay. β-1,3-glucan in RAW264.7 cells was not cytotoxic at any treated concentrations (Figure 1A). The NO production in response to β-1,3-glucan in RAW264.7 was then measured. When cells were treated with different concentrations (50, 100, 250, and 500 μg/mL) of β-1,3-glucan for 24 h, NO production was significant at 250 and 500 μg/mL of β-1,3-glucan compared to the untreated group (untreated 13.90 μM, 250 μg/mL 18.98 μM, 500 μg/mL 19.16 μM), as shown in Figure 1B.

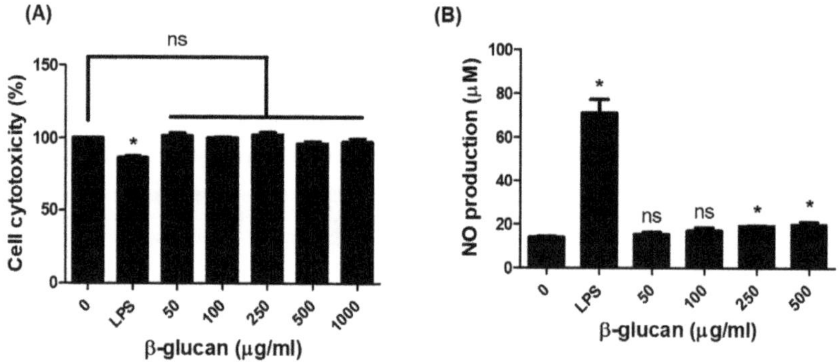

Figure 1. Production of NO metabolites by β-1,3-glucan in RAW264.7 cells. Cells were incubated with a series of concentrations of β-1,3-glucan (0, 50, 100, 250, 500, and 1000 μg/mL) or LPS (1 μg/mL) for 24 h. After the incubation, the (**A**) cytotoxicity by CCK-8 assay and (**B**) NO production in the supernatants collected from the cells by a nitrite/nitrate assay kit were determined. All data are presented as means ± SD, and experiments were performed at least three times. * $p < 0.05$ vs. untreated; ns: not significant.

3.2. Specific Production of Pro-Inflammatory Cytokine TNF-α via a Stimulation of TLR-6 and Dectin-1 Proteins on a Surface of RAW264.7 Cells by β-1,3-Glucan

The production of inflammatory cytokines in macrophages is a hallmark of the innate immune response. Therefore, we investigated the cytokine production triggered by β-1,3-glucan in RAW264.7 cells. For cytokine analysis, the cell-free supernatants were collected from cells treated with β-1,3-glucan for 24 h. Interestingly, β-1,3-glucan significantly stimulated the production of TNF-α (Figure 2A), but not that of IL-6 and IL-1β (Supplementary Figure S1). The presence of β-1,3-glucan significantly increased the expression of TLR6 and dectin-1 on the cell surface (Figure 2B,C), in addition to increasing the expression of pERK and pNF-κB, although not in a concentration-dependent manner.

3.3. Effect of EP on the Weight of Body and Organs in the Immunosuppressed Mice

To determine the immune-enhancing effect of *E. gracilis*, which contains high amounts of β-1,3-glucan in vivo, the immunosuppressed mice induced by intraperitoneal injection of CP (100 mg/kg) were used. Mice received CP on day 1 and day 4 from the first day of oral administration of EP. CP induced a significant decrease in the body weight of mice on day 6 compared to the water-only group (NC) (Figure 3A). By day 8, the mice were in a recovery of body weight except for those in the CP group, and in addition, all EP groups showed a significant difference compared to the CP group (Figure 3B). All the animals were sacrificed after 14 days of oral administration. The liver weight of the mice in the CP group was significantly increased compared with that of the mice in the NC and EP groups, and the spleen weight was also increased (Figure 3D,E). However, the thymus weight did not differ among NC, CP, and RG groups, but was significantly different in EP groups (Figure 3F).

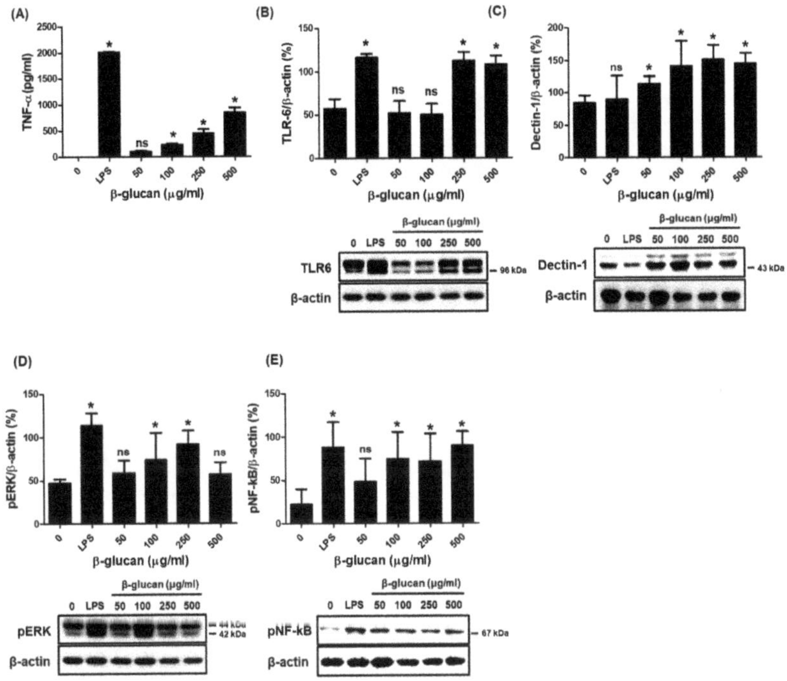

Figure 2. Effect of β-1,3-glucan on TNF-α production and the activation-related proteins in RAW264.7 cells. Cells were incubated with different concentrations (0, 50, 100, 250, and 500 μg/mL) of β-1,3-glucan or LPS for 24 h. The supernatants and cells were then harvested separately for each experiment. (**A**) TNF-α by ELISA assay and the expression of (**B**) TLR-6, (**C**) Dectin-1, (**D**) pERK, and (**E**) pNF-κB by Western blot analysis were identified. All data are presented as means ± SD, and experiments were performed at least three times. * $p < 0.05$ vs. untreated; ns: not significant.

3.4. CBC Analysis of Whole Blood from the Mice Treated with EP

The total white blood cell (WBC) count was lower in all groups treated with CP than in the untreated group (NC), as shown in Figure 4A and Table 1. However, the frequency of myeloid cells (neutrophil; NEU, monocyte; MONO, eosinophil; EOS, basophil; BASO) was relatively increased in the CP-treated groups compared to the untreated group, with the neutrophil level being especially significant (Figure 4B, NEU; NC 14.95%, CP 41.40%, RG 10 mg/kg 37.29%, EP 100 mg/kg 31.99%, EP 300 mg/kg 33.10%, EP 600 mg/kg 36.53%). While the frequency of lymphoid cells (LYM) was significantly reduced in the CP-treated groups compared to the untreated group (NC), it was reduced to a significantly lesser extent in the RG and EP groups (Figure 4C; NC 75.90%, CP 37.20%, RG 10 mg/kg 53.55%, EP 100 mg/kg 56.75%, EP 300 mg/kg 54.00%, EP 600 mg/kg 53.23%). The red blood cell (RBC) count and RDW (%) level of mice in the CP group were significantly different from those in the NC group, but not in the other groups (Figure 4D,E). The platelet (PLT) count was significantly increased in CP-treated mice compared to untreated mice (Figure 4F).

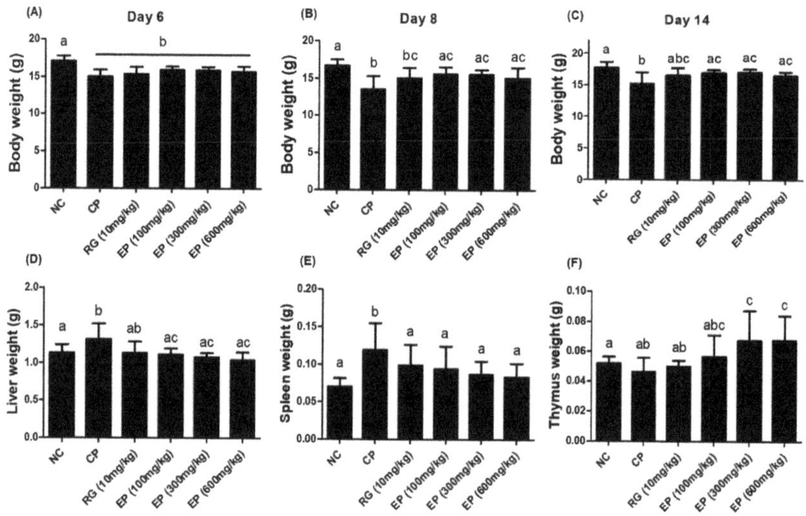

Figure 3. Change in body weight and liver, spleen, and thymus weights of the mice after oral administration of EP. Mice were injected intraperitoneally with CP on days 1 and 4 after starting oral administration of water, RG (10 mg/kg), and three concentrations (100, 300, and 600 mg/kg) of EP, except for the group receiving water only (NC). All specimens were administered orally to the mice for a total of 14 days. (**A–C**) Body weight of mice on days 6, 8, and 14 and the weight of (**D**) liver, (**E**) spleen, and (**F**) thymus isolated from each animal after 14 days of oral administration. All data are presented as means ± SD (n = 8) and analyzed by one-way ANOVA to compare differences between groups. The different letters in the graph indicate a significance between groups, and the *p*-value is less than 0.05.

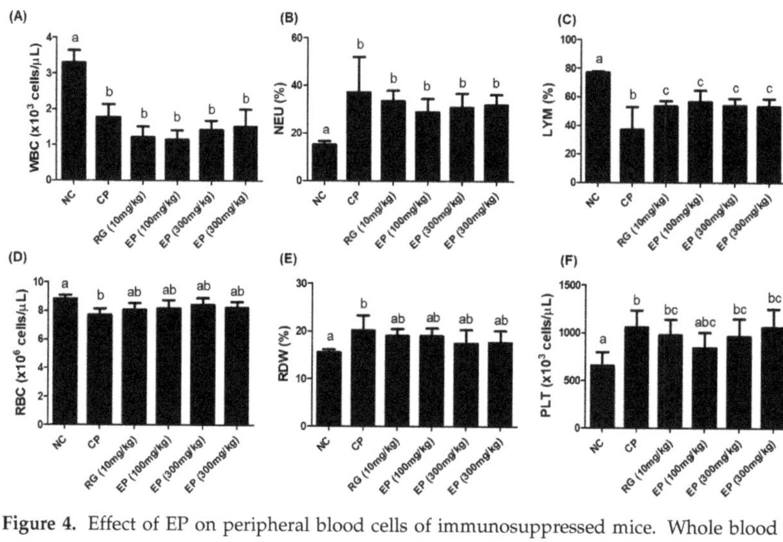

Figure 4. Effect of EP on peripheral blood cells of immunosuppressed mice. Whole blood was collected from mice after oral administration of each sample for 14 days. (**A**) White blood cells (WBC, $\times 10^6$ cells/μL), (**B**) neutrophils (NEU, %), (**C**) lymphocytes (LYM, %), (**D**) red blood cells (RBC, $\times 10^6$ cells/μL), (**E**) red blood cell distribution width (RDW, %), and (**F**) platelets (PLT, $\times 10^3$ cells/μL). All data are presented as means ± SD (n = 8) and analyzed with one-way ANOVA to compare differences between groups. The different letters in the graph indicate a significance between groups, and the *p*-value is less than 0.05.

Table 1. Effect of EP on hematological indices in CP-treated mice.

Hematological Index [1]	Group NC	CP	RG (10 mg/kg)	EP (100 mg/kg)	EP (300 mg/kg)	EP (600 mg/kg)
WBC ($\times 10^3$ cells/μL)	3.40 ± 0.68^{a}	1.68 ± 0.30^{b}	1.48 ± 0.31^{b}	1.12 ± 0.30^{b}	1.34 ± 0.27^{b}	1.52 ± 0.47^{b}
NEU (%)	14.95 ± 2.21^{a}	41.40 ± 17.51^{b}	37.29 ± 8.35^{b}	31.99 ± 7.32^{b}	33.10 ± 6.41^{b}	36.53 ± 10.23^{b}
LYM (%)	75.90 ± 2.18^{a}	37.20 ± 15.88^{b}	53.55 ± 3.64^{c}	56.75 ± 7.83^{c}	54.00 ± 4.96^{c}	55.23 ± 5.54^{c}
MONO (%)	5.97 ± 0.37^{a}	11.17 ± 5.44^{a}	10.08 ± 2.16^{a}	10.36 ± 5.17^{a}	7.84 ± 3.30^{a}	7.96 ± 1.97^{a}
EOS (%)	3.26 ± 1.65^{a}	5.43 ± 5.23^{a}	4.00 ± 3.16^{a}	6.28 ± 2.63^{a}	6.27 ± 4.77^{a}	4.70 ± 3.54^{a}
BASO (%)	0.10 ± 0.00^{a}	0.20 ± 0.15^{a}	0.14 ± 0.07^{a}	0.11 ± 0.04^{a}	0.13 ± 0.05^{a}	0.14 ± 0.07^{a}
RBC ($\times 10^6$ cells/μL)	8.59 ± 0.49^{a}	7.84 ± 0.44^{b}	8.09 ± 0.48^{ab}	8.17 ± 0.46^{ab}	8.26 ± 0.46^{ab}	8.27 ± 0.40^{ab}
HGB (g/dL)	12.83 ± 0.80^{a}	11.41 ± 0.85^{a}	11.76 ± 0.94^{a}	12.24 ± 0.77^{a}	12.04 ± 1.01^{a}	12.03 ± 0.63^{a}
HCT (%)	40.78 ± 3.32^{a}	36.39 ± 3.19^{a}	38.36 ± 1.80^{a}	39.15 ± 1.10^{a}	38.83 ± 1.47^{a}	38.56 ± 1.21^{a}
MCV (fL)	47.46 ± 1.87^{a}	46.44 ± 3.28^{a}	47.55 ± 2.40^{a}	48.05 ± 2.91^{a}	47.08 ± 1.76^{a}	46.78 ± 1.21^{a}
MCH (pg)	14.96 ± 0.1^{a} 4	14.56 ± 0.78^{a}	14.55 ± 0.42^{a}	15.00 ± 0.33^{a}	14.59 ± 0.48^{a}	14.56 ± 0.51^{a}
MCHC (g/dL)	31.56 ± 1.13^{a}	31.43 ± 1.21^{a}	30.64 ± 1.62^{a}	31.29 ± 1.61^{a}	31.04 ± 1.77^{a}	31.18 ± 1.41^{a}
RDW (%)	15.74 ± 0.63^{a}	20.13 ± 3.14^{b}	19.05 ± 1.43^{ab}	19.03 ± 1.61^{ab}	17.48 ± 2.87^{ab}	17.72 ± 2.41^{ab}
MPV (fL)	5.48 ± 0.31^{a}	5.66 ± 0.59^{a}	5.74 ± 0.57^{a}	5.83 ± 0.51^{a}	5.65 ± 0.44^{a}	5.61 ± 0.49^{a}
PLT ($\times 10^3$ cells/μL)	734.5 ± 169.08^{a}	1013.85 ± 177.21^{b}	993.62 ± 161.95^{bc}	845.12 ± 156.75^{abc}	970.25 ± 185.14^{bc}	1073.12 ± 194.64^{bc}

[1] WBC: white blood cells; NEU: neutrophils; LYM: lymphocytes; EOS: eosinophils; BASO: basophils; RBC: red blood cells; HGB: hemoglobin; HCT: hematocrit; MCV: mean corpuscular volume; MCH: mean corpuscular hemoglobin; MCHC: mean corpuscular hemoglobin concentration; RDW: red blood cell distribution width; MPV: mean platelet volume; PLT: platelet count. All data are means ± SD (n = 8) and were analyzed with one-way ANOVA to compare differences between groups. The different letters in the graph indicate a significance between groups, and the *p*-value is less than 0.05.

3.5. Increased Frequency of Lymphoid Cells in Mouse Spleen by EP

The total frequency of lymphocytes in the CBC of CP-treated mice was significantly decreased, but the proliferation of cells isolated from the spleen of mice was not different among all groups (Figure 5A). The frequencies of NK1.1$^+$, CD3$^+$, CD4$^+$, and CD8$^+$ cells were higher in all EP groups than in the others, as shown in Figure 5B–E (NK1.1$^+$: NC 3.3%, CP 6.1%, RG (10 mg/kg) 8.2%, EP (100 mg/kg) 8.9%, EP (300 mg/kg) 9.5%, EP (600 mg/kg) 9.2%; CD3$^+$: NC 32.9%, CP 29.5%, RG (10 mg/kg) 35.5%, EP (100 mg/kg) 35.3%, EP (300 mg/kg) 37.6%, EP (600 mg/kg) 37.9%; CD4$^+$: NC 18.9%, CP 16.4%, RG (10 mg/kg) 21.5%, EP (100 mg/kg) 24.3%, EP (300 mg/kg) 24.9%, EP (600 mg/kg) 27.0%; CD8$^+$: NC 11.6%, CP 10.9%, RG (10 mg/kg) 12.0%, EP (100 mg/kg) 13.3%, EP (300 mg/kg) 15.9%, EP (600 mg/kg) 15.2%). The frequency of B220$^+$ cells was decreased by CP treatment but was significantly restored by RG or EP treatment compared to CP treatment only (Figure 5F; NC 54.3%, CP 21.7%, RG (10 mg/kg) 38.8%, EP (100 mg/kg) 41.4%, EP (300 mg/kg) 41.2%, EP (600 mg/kg) 40.3%).

3.6. Increased Production of Cytokines (TNF-α, IFN-γ, IL-12) and IgM Antibody in Immunosuppressed Mice by EP

The effect of EP on the production of cytokines and antibodies was analyzed in splenocytes or serum of mice by an ELISA assay. The splenocytes isolated from the mouse spleen were treated with or without ConA for 72 h, and then the cell-free supernatants were collected. Cytokines were produced only in the presence of ConA. TNF-α production was significantly increased by treatment with RG or EP compared to the NC group (Figure 6A). The production of IFN-γ and IL-12 cytokines was reduced in CP-treated mice, but it was significantly increased by RG or EP treatment (Figure 6B,C). In addition, the production of IgM antibody in splenocytes of CP-treated mice was low compared to untreated mice with or without ConA, and it was significantly increased by RG or EP treatment compared to CP-treated group (Figure 6D). In the serum, IgM levels were significantly lower with CP treatment but were significantly increased by EP treatment (Figure 6E).

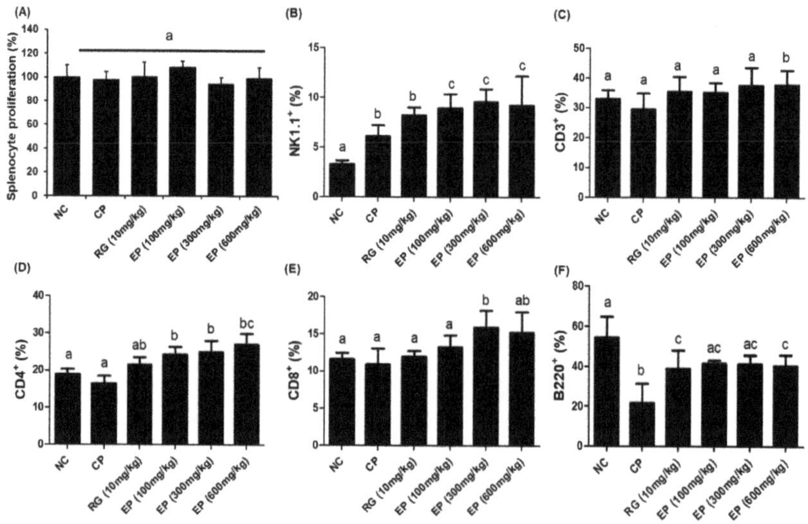

Figure 5. Effect of EP on splenocytes of immunosuppressed mice. (**A**) Splenocyte proliferation by CCK-8 assay and the frequencies of (**B**) NK1.1^{+}, (**C**) CD3^{+}, (**D**) CD4^{+}, (**E**) CD8^{+}, and (**F**) B220^{+} cells by flow cytometry were determined. All results are expressed as means ± SD (n = 8). Data were analyzed by one-way ANOVA to compare differences between groups. The different letters in the graph indicate a significance between groups, and the *p*-value is less than 0.05.

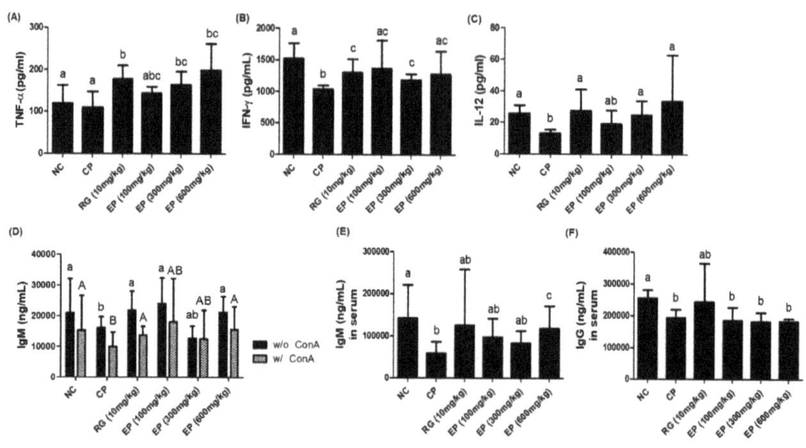

Figure 6. Effect of EP on the production of cytokines and antibodies. Splenocytes isolated from mice were incubated with ConA (10 μg/mL) for 72 h, and the cell-free supernatants were then collected, and mouse serum was separated from whole blood. The levels of cytokines and antibodies were analyzed by ELISA assay kits. The production of (**A**) TNF-α, (**B**) IFN-γ, (**C**) IL-12, and (**D**) IgM in the cell-free supernatants and the levels of (**E**) IgM and (**F**) IgG in the serum were determined. Data were analyzed by one-way ANOVA to compare differences between groups. The different letters in the graph indicate a significance between groups, and the *p*-value is less than 0.05.

3.7. Increased Expression of Dectin-1 in Liver Tissue of Immunosuppressed Mice by EP

In an in vitro study, β-1,3-glucan induced a significant increase in dectin-1 expression in RAW264.7 cells compared to the control (Figure 2E). Therefore, dectin-1 expression in mouse liver tissue was identified by immunohistochemistry (IHC) staining. The expression of dectin-1 was lower in the mouse liver in the CP group than in the untreated group (NC group). RG treatment didn't affect the expression of dectin-1, but EP treatment increased it in a concentration-dependent manner (Figure 7).

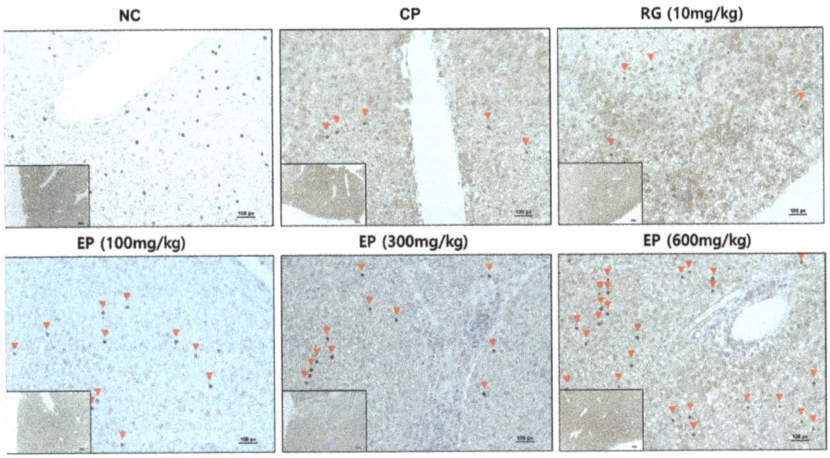

Figure 7. Effect of EP on dectin-1 expression in mouse liver. The liver tissue of mice was collected after 14 days of specimen treatment. The analysis of dectin-1 expression in the liver tissue of mice was performed by immunohistochemistry (IHC) staining. The picture was visualized by light microscopy (40× and 200×). Dectin-1 expression is indicated by black dots, shown by red arrows. The experiment was performed at least three times on different liver tissues from each group, and the upper picture was a representative of all results.

4. Discussion

In this study, the immune-enhancing effect of EP was investigated using CP-induced immunosuppressed mice. *E. gracilis*, a unicellular alga, can accumulate large amounts of β-1,3-glucan (Paramylon) in its cytoplasm [12], which has recently attracted interest for bioproduct development due to its multiple health benefits [25]. β-glucan is a highly conserved group of glucose polymers and is a structural component of various organisms including fungi, algae, bacteria, and plants. Several studies have reported the various biological functions of β-glucan including immunostimulatory, antioxidant, and antitumor effects [10,13,26]. These effects depend on the structure of β-glucan, such as molecular weight, conformation, and modification [27]. Paramylon is a high molecular weight, linear (unbranched) polysaccharide polymer that has recently been explored for product development in many industries due to its unique structure [28]. The immunostimulatory effect of *E. gracilis*, including its paramylon β-glucan, has been reported in several studies, but the biological mechanisms in animals or humans are not yet well understood.

Reactive oxygen species (ROS) and nitric oxide (NO) are redox molecules that serve as key mediators of innate and adaptive immunity. The production of ROS and NO can trigger specific signals in monocytes and participate in the activation of T cells [29]. In porcine leukocytes, only β-glucan from *E. gracilis* and yeast induced ROS production, while other β-glucan (e.g., Laminarin, Scleroglucan) did not [30]. Our study also showed that β-1,3-glucan extracted from *E. gracilis* was able to generate NO metabolites in the mouse macrophage cell RAW264.7 (Figure 1B). NO is synthesized by many immune cells, including macrophages, and triggers inflammatory signals that lead to the secretion of pro-inflammatory cytokines such as TNF-α, IL-1β, IL-6, and IFN-γ [31,32]. RAW264.7 macrophages treated with *E. gracilis*, of which paramylon is a major component, in a concentration-dependent manner secreted TNF-α and IL-6 [33]. Oral administration of paramylon β-1,3-glucan to mice challenged with the influenza virus H1N1 increased survival and cytokine levels (IFN-γ, IL-1β, IL-6, IL-10, and IL-12) compared to untreated mice [34]. This study found that paramylon β-1,3-glucan induced specific production of only TNF-α but not other cytokines (IL-1β, IL-6, and IL-12, not Supplementary Results) in RAW264.7 cells (Figure 2A). Furthermore, treatment of RAW264.7 cells with paramylon β-1,3-glucan (250 and 500 μg/mL) induced the expression of TLR6 and dectin-1 on the cell surface, whereas LPS (1 μg/mL) significantly increased the expression of TLR2/6 on the cell surface (Figure 2B,C, Supplementary Figure S2). Several carbohydrate molecules (e.g., mannan, glucans) bind to pathogen recognition receptors (PRRs) on the surface of immune cells and induce proinflammatory cytokine signaling through the NF-κB and the MAP kinase pathways [35]. Glucans induce an immune response by binding to lectin receptors, one of the PRRs, and in particular, β-glucans recognize detin-1 in cooperation with TLR2 on the surface of macrophages [36]. β-glucan signaling is mediated by multiple receptors that ultimately activate transcription factors such as NF-kB, phospholipase C (PLC), and MAPK [37–39]. Similarly, the binding of paramylon β-1,3-glucan to its receptors increased the expression of pERK and pNF-κB, although not in a concentration-dependent manner (Figure 2D,E).

Cyclophosphamide (CP) is commonly used as an anticancer chemotherapeutic agent, but high doses of CP can cause acute bone marrow depression [23]. When injected into mice, CP can suppress the function of the thymus and spleen. The thymus and spleen are secondary immune organs and are involved in the development of cellular and humoral immunity. C57BL/6 mice injected with CP had decreased body weight, thymus and spleen sizes, and WBC, RBC, and PLT counts [40]. The effect of *E. gracilis* containing its major component on innate and adaptive immune responses has been reported in several studies. In this study, all mice injected with CP lost weight compared to control mice. Interestingly, mice that were orally administered RG and EP lost less weight on day 8 than those that were not (Figure 3B). RG is commonly used in many studies as a positive sample due to its immune-enhancing effects [41]. After 14 days of oral administration, mice were dissected and the weights of the liver, spleen, and thymus were compared, and the weights of the liver and spleen were increased in the CP group compared with the control group. The liver and spleen weights of mice orally administered RG and EP were not significantly different from the control group (Figure 3E,F). Meanwhile, the thymus weight of mice in the CP group was slightly reduced compared with the control. Previously, several studies reported that CP injection decreased the weight of the spleen and thymus in mice [42]; however, the recent observation showed that the change in the weight of the spleen varied according to the dose of CP, but not that of the thymus [40], which was consistent with our results. Interestingly, the thymus of the mice in all EP groups weighed more than that of the mice in the other groups. The total WBC count was reduced in all CP-treated mice compared to controls (Table 1 and Figure 4A), although the frequency of lymphocytes was somewhat restored in mice orally treated with RG and EP and was significantly different from the CP group (Figure 4C). Lymphocytes play an important role in effective defense against infection and control of disease (e.g., cancer) and are involved in homeostasis, where NK, B, and T cells are present [43]. NK cells, belonging to innate immunity, are important lymphocytes because of their ability to directly kill virus-infected or transformed cells and to help other immune cells by producing cytokines such as IFN-γ [3,4,44]. When NK cells encounter virus-infected cells, they produce granules, such as perforin and granzyme B, to induce apoptosis of virus-infected cells [45]. Mice deficient in perforin or IFN-γ could not control viral infection in the spleen and liver [46]. Therefore, in initiating defense against pathogens, the action of NK cells may be very important in the innate and adaptive immune system. A recent study showed that when *E.gracilis* was supplied to healthy subjects for 8 weeks, it enhanced NK activity compared to a group without supplementation [47]. In addition, they reported that the supplementation of *E. gracilis* increased the serum concentration of IFN-γ, IL-2, IL-10, and IL-12 in participants. In this study, EP significantly increased the frequency of $NK1.1^+$ in the spleen of mice compared to other groups of mice (Figure 5B). T lymphocytes, which are involved in cell-mediated immune response, differentiate into the main subtypes, $CD4^+$ T cells, $CD8^+$ T cells, and T regulatory cells [48].

CD4⁺ T cells are helper cells that secrete cytokines, such as IFN-γ, to help activate other cells. CD8⁺ T cells are called effector cells because they can kill infected or transformed cells. The frequency of T lymphocytes (CD3⁺, CD4⁺, CD8⁺) was slightly reduced in the CP group, and the frequency of B220⁺ cells, which represent B lymphocytes, was significantly reduced (Figure 5C–F). Oral administration of EP resulted in relatively higher frequencies of CD3⁺, CD4⁺, and CD8⁺ T cells than no treatment. In addition, the frequency of B220⁺ cells in the spleen of mice in the RG- and EP-treated groups was significantly increased compared with the CP group. Co-inoculation with β-glucan oligosaccharide increases the population of CD4⁺ and CD8⁺ T cells in lymphoid and non-lymphoid tissues of mice immunized with pB144 DNA vaccine [49]. In vivo, ConA stimulation upregulated the mRNA expression of IFN-γ, IL-10, IL-12Rβ1, IL-1β, and IL-2 in spleen cells of β-glucan- or euglena-treated groups [50]. IFN-γ and IL-2 are the major cytokines associated with T-cell activation, with IFN-γ, IL-2, and IL-12 involved in Th1 cell differentiation and IL-4 and IL-10 involved in Th2 cell differentiation [51]. Th1 cells primarily enhance cell-mediated immunity, whereas Th2 cells enhance humoral immunity. This study found that *E. gracilis* powder promoted the secretion of several inflammatory cytokines, including TNF-α, IL-12, and IFN-γ from splenocytes (Figure 6A–C). B lymphocytes are derived from bone marrow and migrate to the spleen, where they develop into mature B cells. When naïve B cells are activated by an antigen (with the help of T_{helper} cells), they proliferate and differentiate into antibody-secreting effector cells (plasma cells). The primary response to an antigen typically produces more IgM than IgG antibodies, and secondary response relatively increases the level of IgG [52]. CP-treated mice had significantly reduced levels of IgM and IgG produced by spleen cells compared to controls (Figure 6D,F). Dietary supplementation with β-1,3-glucan derived from *E. gracilis* increased the levels of IgG, IgM, and IgA in the serum of the animals [53]. In this study, oral administration of EP to mice rescued IgM levels in serum or secreted from splenocytes, but did not affect IgG levels.

Dectin-1 is a C-type lectin receptor found mainly on myeloid cells such as dendritic cells and macrophages, as well as certain lymphoid cells. It acts as a transmembrane recognition receptor (PRR) that specifically binds to various β-1,3-glucans and polysaccharides [54]. When β-1,3-glucans bind to dectin-1 on the surface of dendritic cells or macrophages, it triggers the production of various inflammatory cytokines, including TNF-α, IL-12, and IFN-γ, which enhance adaptive immune responses [13,55]. As noted earlier, β-1,3-glucan derived from *E. gracilis* triggered the specific expression of dectin-1 in mouse macrophage RAW264.7 (Figure 2C). Dectin-1 is broadly expressed on monocytes across different tissues, especially in the liver and lungs [56]. More recently, studies have shown that dectin-1 mRNA expression was suppressed in the liver and lungs of CP-treated mice and that *E. gracilis* provided protection against CP-induced suppression of dectin-1 expression [57], which was consistent with our results (Figure 7). CP significantly decreased the expression of dectin-1 in liver tissues of mice compared to control; however, oral administration of EP restored the expression of dectin-1 in the mouse liver, but this was not observed in RG-treated mice. This result demonstrated that EP could activate the adaptive immune response by inducing the specific expression of dectin-1.

5. Conclusions

This study demonstrated that oral administration of EP to mice helped maintain a high frequency of lymphocytes and upregulate IgM antibody levels through the production of several inflammatory cytokines in CP-induced immunosuppressed mice. In addition, we found that *E. gracilis* induced the specific expression of dectin-1 in mice. Taken together, these results suggest that *E. gracilis* could be used as a potential natural immune stimulator to enhance innate and adaptive immune responses.

Supplementary Materials: The following supporting information can be downloaded at: https://www.mdpi.com/article/10.3390/nu16183158/s1; Figure S1: Inflammatory cytokines produced by RAW264.7 cells treated with β-1,3-glucan; Figure S2: Expression of TLR2 and TLR4 in RAW264.7 cells treated with β-1,3-glucan; Figure S3: Changes in the spleen and thymus of EP-treated mice.

Author Contributions: Conceptualization, H.H.L. and H.C.; methodology, H.H.L. and H.C.; formal analysis, H.H.L., J.-Y.S. and H.C.; investigation, H.H.L. and J.-Y.S.; resources, H.K. and H.C.; data curation, H.H.L. and H.C.; writing—original draft preparation, H.H.L. and H.C.; writing—review and editing, H.K. and H.C.; funding acquisition, H.K. and H.C. All authors have read and agreed to the published version of the manuscript.

Funding: This research was funded by JUYEONG NS Co., Ltd. (202400020001) and supported by the Priority Research Center Program through the NRF, funded by the Korean Ministry of Education, Science and Technology (2016R1A6A1A03007648), as well as a grant from the Korean Government (MSIT) (2020R1A5A2017323).

Institutional Review Board Statement: The study was conducted according to the guidelines of the Declaration of Helsinki and approved by the animal experiments committee of Duksung Women's University (permit No. 2024-004-026, May 2024).

Informed Consent Statement: Not applicable.

Data Availability Statement: All the data are contained within the article.

Conflicts of Interest: The authors declare no conflicts of interest.

References

1. Tubo, N.J.; Jenkins, M.K. CD4$^+$ T Cells: Guardians of the phagosome. *Clin. Microbiol. Rev.* **2014**, *27*, 200–213. [CrossRef] [PubMed]
2. Grégoire, C.; Chasson, L.; Luci, C.; Tomasello, E.; Geissmann, F.; Vivier, E.; Walzer, T. The trafficking of natural killer cells. *Immunol. Rev.* **2007**, *220*, 169–182. [CrossRef] [PubMed]
3. Martínez-Lostao, L.; Anel, A.; Pardo, J. How Do Cytotoxic Lymphocytes Kill Cancer Cells? *Clin. Cancer Res. Off. J. Am. Assoc. Cancer Res.* **2015**, *21*, 5047–5056. [CrossRef] [PubMed]
4. Fauriat, C.; Long, E.O.; Ljunggren, H.G.; Bryceson, Y.T. Regulation of human NK-cell cytokine and chemokine production by target cell recognition. *Blood* **2010**, *115*, 2167–2176. [CrossRef]
5. Janeway, C.A., Jr.; Travers, P.; Walport, M.; Shlomchik, M. Immunobiology: The Immune System in Health and Disease. In *Principles of Innate and Adaptive Immunity*, 5th ed.; Garland Science: New York, NY, USA, 2001.
6. Palacios-Pedrero, M.; Osterhaus, A.; Becker, T.; Elbahesh, H.; Rimmelzwaan, G.F.; Saletti, G. Aging and Options to Halt Declining Immunity to Virus Infections. *Front. Immunol.* **2021**, *12*, 681449. [CrossRef]
7. Chae, S.R.; Hwang, E.J.; Shin, H.S. Single cell protein production of *Euglena gracilis* and carbon dioxide fixation in an innovative photo-bioreactor. *Bioresour. Technol.* **2006**, *97*, 322–329. [CrossRef]
8. Ivušić, F.; Rezić, T.; Šantek, B. Heterotrophic Cultivation of *Euglena gracilis* in Stirred Tank Bioreactor: A Promising Bioprocess for Sustainable Paramylon Production. *Molecules* **2022**, *27*, 5866. [CrossRef]
9. Takeyama, H.; Kanamaru, A.; Yoshino, Y.; Kakuta, H.; Kawamura, Y.; Matsunaga, T. Production of antioxidant vitamins, β-carotene, vitamin C, and vitamin E, by two-step culture of *Euglena gracilis* Z. *Biotechnol. Bioeng.* **1997**, *53*, 185–190. [CrossRef]
10. Rodríguez Zavala, J.S.; Ortiz Cruz, M.A.; Mendoza Hernández, G.; Moreno Sánchez, R. Increased synthesis of α-tocopherol, paramylon and tyrosine by *Euglena gracilis* under conditions of high biomass production. *J. Appl. Microbiol.* **2010**, *109*, 2160–2172. [CrossRef]
11. Pollak, D.W.; Bostick, M.W.; Yoon, H.; Wang, J.; Hollerbach, D.H.; He, H.; Damude, H.G.; Zhang, H.; Yadav, N.S.; Hong, S.-P.; et al. Isolation of a Δ5 Desaturase Gene from *Euglena gracilis* and Functional Dissection of Its HPGG and HDASH Motifs. *Lipids* **2012**, *47*, 913–926. [CrossRef]
12. Barsanti, L.; Vismara, R.; Passarelli, V.; Gualtieri, P. Paramylon (β-1,3-glucan) content in wild type and WZSL mutant of *Euglena gracilis*. Effects of growth conditions. *J. Appl. Phycol.* **2001**, *13*, 59–65. [CrossRef]
13. Russo, R.; Barsanti, L.; Evangelista, V.; Frassanito, A.M.; Longo, V.; Pucci, L.; Penno, G.; Gualtieri, P. *Euglena gracilis* paramylon activates human lymphocytes by upregulating pro-inflammatory factors. *Food Sci. Nutr.* **2017**, *5*, 205–214. [CrossRef]
14. C.Ooi, E.V.; Liu, F. Immunomodulation and Anti-Cancer Activity of Polysaccharide-Protein Complexes. *Curr. Med. Chem.* **2000**, *7*, 715–729. [CrossRef]
15. Gissibl, A.; Care, A.; Parker, L.M.; Iqbal, S.; Hobba, G.; Nevalainen, H.; Sunna, A. Microwave pretreatment of paramylon enhances the enzymatic production of soluble β-1,3-glucans with immunostimulatory activity. *Carbohydr. Polym.* **2018**, *196*, 339–347. [CrossRef] [PubMed]
16. Patidar, A.; Mahanty, T.; Raybarman, C.; Sarode, A.Y.; Basak, S.; Saha, B.; Bhattacharjee, S. Barley beta-Glucan and Zymosan induce Dectin-1 and Toll-like receptor 2 co-localization and anti-leishmanial immune response in Leishmania donovani-infected BALB/c mice. *Scand. J. Immunol.* **2020**, *92*, e12952. [CrossRef]
17. Brown, G.D. Dectin-1: A signalling non-TLR pattern-recognition receptor. *Nat. Rev. Immunol.* **2006**, *6*, 33–43. [CrossRef] [PubMed]

18. Brown, G.D.; Herre, J.; Williams, D.L.; Willment, J.A.; Marshall, A.S.; Gordon, S. Dectin-1 mediates the biological effects of beta-glucans. *J. Exp. Med.* **2003**, *197*, 1119–1124. [CrossRef]
19. Underhill, D.M.; Rossnagle, E.; Lowell, C.A.; Simmons, R.M. Dectin-1 activates Syk tyrosine kinase in a dynamic subset of macrophages for reactive oxygen production. *Blood* **2005**, *106*, 2543–2550. [CrossRef]
20. Galluzzi, L.; Buqué, A.; Kepp, O.; Zitvogel, L.; Kroemer, G. Immunological Effects of Conventional Chemotherapy and Targeted Anticancer Agents. *Cancer Cell* **2015**, *28*, 690–714. [CrossRef]
21. Bao, L.; Hao, C.; Wang, J.; Wang, D.; Zhao, Y.; Li, Y.; Yao, W. High-Dose Cyclophosphamide Administration Orchestrates Phenotypic and Functional Alterations of Immature Dendritic Cells and Regulates Th Cell Polarization. *Front. Pharmacol.* **2020**, *11*, 00775. [CrossRef]
22. Mills, K.A.; Chess-Williams, R.; McDermott, C. Novel insights into the mechanism of cyclophosphamide-induced bladder toxicity: Chloroacetaldehyde's contribution to urothelial dysfunction in vitro. *Arch. Toxicol.* **2019**, *93*, 3291–3303. [CrossRef] [PubMed]
23. Lee, H.H.; Cho, Y.; Kim, G.H.; Cho, H. Undaria pinnatifida Fucoidan-Rich Extract Recovers Immunity of Immunosuppressed Mice. *J. Microbiol. Biotechnol.* **2020**, *30*, 439–447. [CrossRef]
24. Kim, S.; Lee, H.H.; Kang, C.H.; Kang, H.; Cho, H. Immune-Enhancing Effects of Limosilactobacillus fermentum in BALB/c Mice Immunosuppressed by Cyclophosphamide. *Nutrients* **2023**, *15*, 1038. [CrossRef] [PubMed]
25. Nakashima, A.; Yamada, K.; Iwata, O.; Sugimoto, R.; Atsuji, K.; Ogawa, T.; Ishibashi-Ohgo, N.; Suzuki, K. β-Glucan in Foods and Its Physiological Functions. *J. Nutr. Sci. Vitaminol.* **2018**, *64*, 8–17. [CrossRef] [PubMed]
26. Isoda, N.; Eguchi, Y.; Nukaya, H.; Hosho, K.; Suga, Y.; Suga, T.; Nakazawa, S.; Sugano, K. Clinical efficacy of superfine dispersed lentinan (beta-1,3-glucan) in patients with hepatocellular carcinoma. *Hepato-Gastroenterology* **2009**, *56*, 437–441.
27. Rahar, S.; Swami, G.; Nagpal, N.; Nagpal, M.A.; Singh, G.S. Preparation, characterization, and biological properties of β-glucans. *J. Adv. Pharm. Technol. Res.* **2011**, *2*, 94–103. [CrossRef]
28. Gissibl, A.; Sun, A.; Care, A.; Nevalainen, H.; Sunna, A. Bioproducts From *Euglena gracilis*: Synthesis and Applications. *Front. Bioeng. Biotechnol.* **2019**, *7*, 108. [CrossRef]
29. Wink, D.A.; Hines, H.B.; Cheng, R.Y.; Switzer, C.H.; Flores-Santana, W.; Vitek, M.P.; Ridnour, L.A.; Colton, C.A. Nitric oxide and redox mechanisms in the immune response. *J. Leukoc. Biol.* **2011**, *89*, 873–891. [CrossRef]
30. Sonck, E.; Stuyven, E.; Goddeeris, B.; Cox, E. The effect of beta-glucans on porcine leukocytes. *Vet. Immunol. Immunopathol.* **2010**, *135*, 199–207. [CrossRef]
31. Turpaev, K.; Glatigny, A.; Bignon, J.; Delacroix, H.; Drapier, J.C. Variation in gene expression profiles of human monocytic U937 cells exposed to various fluxes of nitric oxide. *Free Radic. Biol. Med.* **2010**, *48*, 298–305. [CrossRef]
32. Liu, T.; Zhang, L.; Joo, D.; Sun, S.-C. NF-κB signaling in inflammation. *Signal Transduct. Target. Ther.* **2017**, *2*, 17023. [CrossRef]
33. Guo, Q.; Bi, D.; Wu, M.; Yu, B.; Hu, L.; Liu, C.; Gu, L.; Zhu, H.; Lei, A.; Xu, X.; et al. Immune activation of murine RAW264.7 macrophages by sonicated and alkalized paramylon from *Euglena gracilis*. *BMC Microbiol.* **2020**, *20*, 171. [CrossRef] [PubMed]
34. Nakashima, A.; Suzuki, K.; Asayama, Y.; Konno, M.; Saito, K.; Yamazaki, N.; Takimoto, H. Oral administration of *Euglena gracilis* Z and its carbohydrate storage substance provides survival protection against influenza virus infection in mice. *Biochem. Biophys. Res. Commun.* **2017**, *494*, 379–383. [CrossRef] [PubMed]
35. Mazgaeen, L.; Gurung, P. Recent Advances in Lipopolysaccharide Recognition Systems. *Int. J. Mol. Sci.* **2020**, *21*, 379. [CrossRef] [PubMed]
36. Yadav, M.; Schorey, J.S. The beta-glucan receptor dectin-1 functions together with TLR2 to mediate macrophage activation by mycobacteria. *Blood* **2006**, *108*, 3168–3175. [CrossRef]
37. Dennehy, K.M.; Ferwerda, G.; Faro-Trindade, I.; Pyz, E.; Willment, J.A.; Taylor, P.R.; Kerrigan, A.; Tsoni, S.V.; Gordon, S.; Meyer-Wentrup, F.; et al. Syk kinase is required for collaborative cytokine production induced through Dectin-1 and Toll-like receptors. *Eur. J. Immunol.* **2008**, *38*, 500–506. [CrossRef]
38. Choi, E.Y.; Lee, S.S.; Hyeon, J.Y.; Choe, S.H.; Keum, B.R.; Lim, J.M.; Park, D.C.; Choi, I.S.; Cho, K.K. Effects of β-Glucan on the Release of Nitric Oxide by Macrophages Stimulated with Lipopolysaccharide. *Asian-Australas. J. Anim. Sci.* **2016**, *29*, 1664–1674. [CrossRef] [PubMed]
39. Batbayar, S.; Lee, D.H.; Kim, H.W. Immunomodulation of Fungal β-Glucan in Host Defense Signaling by Dectin-1. *Biomol. Ther.* **2012**, *20*, 433–445. [CrossRef]
40. Feng, L.; Huang, Q.; Huang, Z.; Li, H.; Qi, X.; Wang, Y.; Liu, Z.; Liu, X.; Lu, L. Optimized Animal Model of Cyclophosphamide-induced Bone Marrow Suppression. *Basic Clin. Pharmacol. Toxicol.* **2016**, *119*, 428–435. [CrossRef]
41. Hyun, S.H.; Ahn, H.Y.; Kim, H.J.; Kim, S.W.; So, S.H.; In, G.; Park, C.K.; Han, C.K. Immuno-enhancement effects of Korean Red Ginseng in healthy adults: A randomized, double-blind, placebo-controlled trial. *J. Ginseng Res.* **2021**, *45*, 191–198. [CrossRef]
42. Zhao, N.; Wang, L.; Mou, H.Y.; Liang, M.; Yue, W. Synergism and attenuation effects of taurine on cyclophosphamide. *Ai Zheng = Aizheng = Chin. J. Cancer* **2009**, *28*, 244–248.
43. Arango-Prado, M.D.C.; Villegas-Valverde, C.A.; Torres-López, G.; Soto-Pardeiro, P.; Suárez-Reyes, A.; Faxas-García, M.E.; Diéguez-Rodríguez, V.; Gracia-Medina, E.; Esperón-Noa, R.; Del Castillo-Bahi, R.; et al. Lymphocyte Subsets in Defense Against New Pathogens in Patients with Cancer. *MEDICC Rev.* **2022**, *24*, 26–34. [CrossRef] [PubMed]
44. Lodoen, M.B.; Lanier, L.L. Natural killer cells as an initial defense against pathogens. *Curr. Opin. Immunol.* **2006**, *18*, 391–398. [CrossRef]

45. Osińska, I.; Popko, K.; Demkow, U. Perforin: An important player in immune response. *Cent.-Eur. J. Immunol.* **2014**, *39*, 109–115. [CrossRef]
46. Loh, J.; Chu, D.T.; O'Guin, A.K.; Yokoyama, W.M.; Virgin, H.W.T. Natural killer cells utilize both perforin and gamma interferon to regulate murine cytomegalovirus infection in the spleen and liver. *J. Virol.* **2005**, *79*, 661–667. [CrossRef]
47. Park, S.-y.; Kim, K.J.; Jo, S.M.; Jeon, J.-Y.; Kim, B.-R.; Hwang, J.E.; Kim, J.Y. *Euglena gracilis* (Euglena) powder supplementation enhanced immune function through natural killer cell activity in apparently healthy participants: A randomized, double-blind, placebo-controlled trial. *Nutr. Res.* **2023**, *119*, 90–97. [CrossRef] [PubMed]
48. Sauls, R.S.; McCausland, C.; Taylor, B.N. Histology, T-Cell Lymphocyte. In *StatPearls*; StatPearls Publishing: Treasure Island, FL, USA, 2024.
49. Wang, J.; Dong, S.; Liu, C.; Wang, W.; Sun, S.; Gu, J.; Wang, Y.; Boraschi, D.; Qu, D. β-Glucan oligosaccharide enhances $CD8^+$ T cells immune response induced by a DNA vaccine encoding hepatitis B virus core antigen. *J. Biomed. Biotechnol.* **2010**, *2010*, 645213. [CrossRef]
50. Jo, K.A.; Kim, K.J.; Park, S.Y.; Jeon, J.Y.; Hwang, J.E.; Kim, J.Y. Evaluation of the Effects of *Euglena gracilis* on Enhancing Immune Responses in RAW264.7 Cells and a Cyclophosphamide-Induced Mouse Model. *J. Microbiol. Biotechnol.* **2023**, *33*, 493–499. [CrossRef]
51. Lee, G.R. Molecular Mechanisms of T Helper Cell Differentiation and Functional Specialization. *Immune Netw.* **2023**, *23*, e4. [CrossRef]
52. Bandilla, K.K.; McDuffie, F.C.; Gleich, G.J. Immunoglobulin classes of antibodies produced in the primary and secondary responses in man. *Clin. Exp. Immunol.* **1969**, *5*, 627–641.
53. de Carvalho, R.H.; Callegari, M.A.; Dias, C.P.; Kirwan, S.; da Costa, M.C.R.; da Silva, C.A. *Euglena gracilis* β-Glucans (1,3): Enriching Colostrum of Sow for Enhanced Piglet Immunity. *Animals* **2023**, *13*, 3490. [CrossRef] [PubMed]
54. Brown, G.D.; Gordon, S. A new receptor for β-glucans. *Nature* **2001**, *413*, 36–37. [CrossRef] [PubMed]
55. Barsanti, L.; Gualtieri, P. Paramylon, a Potent Immunomodulator from WZSL Mutant of *Euglena gracilis*. *Molecules* **2019**, *24*, 3114. [CrossRef] [PubMed]
56. Herre, J.; Gordon, S.; Brown, G.D. Dectin-1 and its role in the recognition of β-glucans by macrophages. *Mol. Immunol.* **2004**, *40*, 869–876. [CrossRef]
57. Yang, H.; Choi, K.; Kim, K.J.; Park, S.Y.; Jeon, J.Y.; Kim, B.G.; Kim, J.Y. Immunoenhancing Effects of *Euglena gracilis* on a Cyclophosphamide-Induced Immunosuppressive Mouse Model. *J. Microbiol. Biotechnol.* **2022**, *32*, 228–237. [CrossRef]

nutrients

MDPI

Article

Capsaicin Improves Systemic Inflammation, Atherosclerosis, and Macrophage-Derived Foam Cells by Stimulating PPAR Gamma and TRPV1 Receptors

Danielle Lima Ávila [1], Weslley Fernandes-Braga [1,†], Janayne Luihan Silva [1], Elandia Aparecida Santos [1], Gianne Campos [2], Paola Caroline Lacerda Leocádio [1], Luciano Santos Aggum Capettini [2], Edenil Costa Aguilar [1,†] and Jacqueline Isaura Alvarez-Leite [1,*]

1 Departamento de Bioquímica e Imunologia, ICB, Universidade Federal de Minas Gerais, Belo Horizonte 31270-901, Brazil; danilimavila@gmail.com (D.L.Á.); weslley.fernandes.braga@gmail.com (W.F.-B.); janayneluihan@gmail.com (J.L.S.); elandianutri@gmail.com (E.A.S.); paolaleocadio@yahoo.com.br (P.C.L.L.); edenilaguilar@gmail.com (E.C.A.)

2 Departamento de Farmacologia, ICB, Universidade Federal de Minas Gerais, Belo Horizonte 31270-901, Brazil; giannepcampos@gmail.com (G.C.); lucianocapettini@gmail.com (L.S.A.C.)

* Correspondence: alvarez@ufmg.br

† Current address: Department of Immunology and Immunotherapy, Icahn School of Medicine at Mount Sinai (ISMMS), New York, NY 10029, USA.

Abstract: Background: Capsaicin, a bioactive compound found in peppers, is recognized for its anti-inflammatory, antioxidant, and anti-lipidemic properties. This study aimed to evaluate the effects of capsaicin on atherosclerosis progression. Methods: Apolipoprotein E knockout mice and their C57BL/6 controls were utilized to assess blood lipid profile, inflammatory status, and atherosclerotic lesions. We also examined the influence of capsaicin on cholesterol influx and efflux, and the role of TRPV1 and PPARγ signaling pathways in bone marrow-derived macrophages. Results: Capsaicin treatment reduced weight gain, visceral adiposity, blood triglycerides, and total and non-HDL cholesterol. These improvements were associated with a reduction in atherosclerotic lesions in the aorta and carotid. Capsaicin also improved hepatic oxidative and inflammatory status. Systemic inflammation was also reduced, as indicated by reduced leukocyte rolling and adhesion on the mesenteric plexus. Capsaicin decreased foam cell formation by reducing cholesterol influx through scavenger receptor A and increasing cholesterol efflux via ATP-binding cassette transporter A1, an effect primarily linked to TRPV1 activation. Conclusions: These findings underscore the potential of capsaicin as a promising agent for atherosclerosis prevention, highlighting its comprehensive role in modulating lipid metabolism, foam cell formation, and inflammatory responses.

Keywords: atherosclerosis; capsaicin; foam cells; inflammation; TRPV1; PPARγ

1. Introduction

Capsaicin (trans-8-methyl-*N*-vanillyl-6-nonenamide, C18H27NO3) is a prominent member of the capsaicinoids, a group of lipophilic and volatile compounds. Capsaicin (Cap) is the most pungent and abundant among the capsaicinoids [1]. The vanilloid ring in Cap has a high affinity for the transient receptor potential vanilloid subtype 1 (TRPV1), a non-selective cation channel widely distributed in various tissues. This receptor is highly expressed in neural and adipose tissue, hepatocytes, leukocytes, and endothelial cells [2]. As a polymodal receptor, TRPV1 responds to a broad spectrum of physical and chemical stimuli, with Cap being its primary exogenous ligand.

For decades, Cap has been extensively studied as an adjuvant for treating inflammatory diseases, particularly neuropathic pain. More recently, the potential effects of Cap on chronic non-communicable diseases have gained interest [3].

Capsaicin's biological activities include analgesic, anesthetic, anti-inflammatory, antioxidant, and thermogenic effects, which are potentially beneficial in chronic diseases such as obesity, systemic arterial hypertension, diabetes mellitus, and dyslipidemias [4–7].

Regarding atherosclerosis, capsaicin intake can improve lipid profiles, reduce inflammation, and mitigate endothelial dysfunction, all of which are crucial factors in preventing or slowing the progression of atherosclerosis [8]. Therefore, our objective was to evaluate the role of Cap on risk factors associated with atherosclerosis using ApoE KO mice, a model highly susceptible to atherosclerosis. Specifically, we focused on its effects on plaque formation as well as its role in regulating intracellular cholesterol in macrophage-derived foam cells.

2. Materials and Methods

2.1. *In Vivo Study*

Forty 6–8 week-old female mice deficient in the apoprotein E (ApoE KO) and their wild type (WT) C57BL/6 controls (n = 18), originally from Jackson Laboratory and kept in the animal facility of the Federal University of Minas Gerais (Belo Horizonte, Brazil), were divided according to initial body weight into groups. The WT and ApoE-KO groups received a standard diet (AIN-96M) supplemented with 0.75% cholesterol, and WT + Cap and ApoE + Cap groups received the same diet supplemented with 0.015% Cap (Sigma, Ronkonkoma, NY, USA), as previously described [9,10]. Animals had ad libitum access to water and food, and were maintained under controlled conditions (temperature: 26–28 °C, light-dark cycles: 12 h) in collective cages (2–3 mice/cage) within the same animal facility room. Mice were housed in cages that were clearly labeled with the corresponding descriptions of their respective experimental groups to mitigate any potential dietary contamination. In the third week of the diet, animals underwent carotid occlusion surgery to accelerate atherosclerotic development. In the fifth experimental week, after overnight fasting, animals were anesthetized for blood collection and euthanized by exsanguination. Following perfusion with phosphate-buffered saline (PBS), liver, aorta, and carotid samples were collected. Weekly assessments included body weight and food intake for energy consumption and weight gain calculations. Liver and visceral adipose tissue weight were measured to calculate relative weight (tissue/body weight × 100). Biological samples were assigned unique codes to ensure that the researchers remained blinded to the specific group assignments of the samples, thereby preserving the integrity of the experimental design and minimizing bias in the analysis. This study was approved by the Ethics Committee of Animal Experimentation—UFMG (# 232/2016). Mice that presented any health issues (such as malocclusion due to incisors overgrowth) were excluded.

2.1.1. Carotid Obstruction Surgery

Carotid obstruction was performed to accelerate atherosclerosis formation. The surgery procedure followed the method described by Nam et al. [11]. Briefly, animals were anesthetized (ketamine 80 mg/kg, xylazine 15 mg/kg) and maintained on a thermal blanket at 37 °C. The left carotid artery was exposed and delicately tied with surgical wire (Sil Silkam 3/0, B. Braun, Germany). Afterward, the region was sutured, and the mice were observed until complete recovery.

2.1.2. Biochemical Determinations

Blood glucose, total cholesterol (TC), HDL cholesterol (HDL-c), and triglycerides (TG) were quantified using colorimetric assay kits (Labtest, Lagoa Santa, Brazil) and following the manufacturer's recommendations. The atherogenic fraction, non-HDL cholesterol (non-HDLc), was calculated from the difference between TC and HDL-c.

2.1.3. Quantification of the Atherosclerosis Area

The aortas were removed, cleaned, and stained with SUDAN IV, as previously described [12]. Image acquisition and analysis were performed using the Image-Pro Plus version 6.3 analyzer (Image-Pro Plus Software, Rockville, MD, USA). The results were presented as the percentage of the aorta area affected by fatty streak. Carotids were included in the Tissue Freezing Medium (Jung Tissue Freezing Medium; Leica Microsystems, Wetzlar, Germany) and were immediately frozen. After processing, slides were stained with Hematoxylin-Eosin (HE) for analysis using Image-Pro Plus software.

2.1.4. Immunofluorescence

The carotid slides were fixed in acetone, permeabilized, and blocked with 0.1% Triton X-100 and 4% BSA in PBS for 1 h before overnight incubation with the primary antibodies (mouse CD36 anti-mouse, Santa Cruz, Dallas, TX, USA; rat MOMA anti-mouse, Bio-Rad Hercules, CA, USA diluted 1:200). After washing, slides were incubated with fluorescent secondary antibodies (rabbit FITC anti-mouse—Santa Cruz; goat Alexa Fluoride 647 anti-mouse—BD Pharmigen, San Diego, CA, USA) for 2 h, washed and covered with DAPI-containing mounting medium. The images were captured with a Nikon Eclipse Ti fluorescence microscope (Melville, NY, USA), and the intraplaque fluorescence intensity (FI) was analyzed using the ImageJ software 1.39. The content of CD36 and MOMA in the lesion was expressed as the fluorescence intensity (FI).

2.1.5. Determination of NAG and MPO Activities

N-acetyl-beta-D-glucosaminidase (NAG) and myeloperoxidase (MPO) activities were measured to assess macrophage and neutrophil infiltrations, respectively, as previously described [13].

2.1.6. Cytokine Determination

To evaluate inflammatory status, TNF and IFN-γ, IL-6, and IL-10 concentrations were detected in liver homogenate by ELISA using a commercial kit (Biolegend, San Diego, CA, USA) and following the manufacturer's instructions.

2.1.7. Intravital Microscopy of Mesenteric Plexus

Intravital microscopy was performed as described [14] to evaluate inflammation in an in vivo real-time manner. Mice were kept in a thermal blanket (37 °C) throughout the procedure. After anesthesia, animals were injected (IV) with 0.1 mL of Rhodamine 6 G (0.5 mg/mL) (Sigma Aldrich, St. Louis, MI, USA) for fluorescence visualization of leukocytes in mesenteric microcirculation. Afterward, the abdominal region was opened, and the intestinal loops were exposed for the mesenteric microcirculation visualization using a microscope Apotome 2 (Zeiss, Oberkochen, Germany) with a 100 × increase. Video captures were made for 10 min for each animal. The number of rolling or adhered cells was counted by delimiting an area in the vessel lumen of 200 μm × 250 μm for 1 min for each count. Cells remaining in the same place in the delimited area for at least 30 s were considered adhered. All analyses were performed in triplicate using the ZEN Blue software 2.1 (Zeiss). The results were expressed as the number of rolling cells or the number of adhered cells/min. After data acquisition, animals were euthanized under anesthesia, as described above.

2.2. *In Vitro Studies*

2.2.1. Preparation of Dil-Oxldl

Native human LDL was isolated by gradient ultracentrifugation from the plasma of healthy donors and was isolated as described by Chung and colleagues [15]. LDL protein concentration was then determined by Lowry et al. [16]. LDL was labeled with DiI as previously described [17]. A solution of 1,1′-Dioctadecyl-3,3,3′,3′-tetramethylindocarbocyanine perchlorate (Dil, Sigma-Aldrich, USA) was prepared by mixing DiI 3 mg/mL of DMSO. This solution was added to the LDL (50 μL of Dil solution for each mg of LDL), followed by overnight incubation at 37 °C in the dark. After incubation, the labeled LDL was reisolated by ultracentrifugation, dialyzed against PBS, and filter sterilized as described above. The oxLDL-Dil preparation was carried out as described by Fernandes-Braga et al. [18]. Dil-LDL oxidation was obtained by incubation with 10 mM $CuSO_4$ for 24 h at 4 °C in the dark. The oxidation was stopped by adding 0.5 M EDTA solution at a final concentration of 0.24 mM. Dil-oxLDL was subjected to new ultracentrifugation (50,000 rpm, 2:30 hs), new dialysis for 24 h, and filtration (0.22 μM) before use.

2.2.2. Cell Cultures

Bone marrow-derived macrophage (BMDM): Cells were extracted in a sterile environment from bone marrow that was derived from the femur and tibia of C57BL/6 mice and deposited in an ice-cold Falcon tube containing RPMI medium without fetal bovine serum (FBS). After centrifugation at 200× *g* for 10 min at 40 °C, cells were resuspended in RPMI for differentiation into macrophages in a 5% CO_2 atmosphere, at 37 °C, for 7 days, changing the medium on the 4th day. The cells were washed, and the adhered macrophages were released by ice-cold 10 mM EDTA solution. The released macrophages were placed in an RPMI medium supplemented with 5% FBS for experimental cultures.

2.2.3. Solutions for Cell Cultures

The Capsaicin used was as follows: Cap stock solution at a concentration of 1 mM (*N*-vanillylnonanamide—Capsaicin—Sigma-Aldrich, purity ≥ 97%) diluted in 1.8% NaCl and ethanol, in a 1:1 ratio. This solution was then filtered through a 0.22 μm sterile filter and stored at 4 °C for up to 90 days.

Capsazepine (CZE) was diluted in DMSO to a final concentration of 1 mM (stock solution), filtered through a sterile 0.22 μm filter, and stored at −20 °C for up to 30 days. The concentration used in the tests was 10 μM, as previously described [19,20].

GW9662: The solution of the irreversible and selective PPARγ antagonist, GW9662 (Santa Cruz), was diluted to a concentration of 0.1 mM in DMSO. The solution was filtered (0.22 μm sterile filter) and stored at −20 °C for up to 60 days. The concentration used in the tests was 5 μM, as previously described [21,22].

Flow cytometry. The uptake of oxLDL-Dil, as well as the expression of the influx scavenger receptors CD36 and SRA, and those of efflux, ABCA1, and ABCG1, were detected on the macrophage surface by flow cytometry.

Cells were seeded in round-bottom 96-well plates with 5×10^5 cells/well, in their respective medium supplemented with 5% SBF, to provide a minimum amount of HDL to enable cholesterol efflux.

Cells were pre-incubated without inhibitor or with 10 μM Capsazepine (TRPV1 antagonist) or 5 μM of GW9662 (PPARγ antagonist) for 1 h. After washing, the cells were then incubated with 1 μM or 5 μM of Cap for 2 h. After new washing to remove Cap, cells were incubated with oxLDL-Dil (final concentration of 50 μg/mL) for 4 h. Afterward, the cells were centrifuged and incubated for 30 min at room temperature with one of the following primary antibodies: mouse antimouse-CD36 (Santa Cruz, Dallas, TX, USA); goat antimouse SR-A (Santa Cruz); mouse antimouse-ABCA1 (Novus Biologicals, Centennial, CO, USA); or rabbit antimouse-ABCG1 (Novus Biologicals, Centennial, CO, USA). Cells were washed twice with PBS Wash before secondary antibodies were incubated for 30 min according to the primary antibody: goat anti-mouse Alexa Fluor 647 (Cell Signaling, Danvers, MA, USA), rabbit anti-goat Alexa 647, and donkey anti-rabbit CFL 647 (Santa Cruz). In the end, the cells were washed and fixed with 2% paraformaldehyde/PBS for 30 min at room temperature for subsequent readings on a FACS CaliburTM cytometer, using the FL-2 and FL-4 filters for Dil and the Alexa 647 probes, respectively. Data acquisition was carried out using the BD CellQuest Pro software 5.0.1, and the delimitation of the cell population was carried out using the size and internal complexity parameters (FSC and SSC parameters, respectively). Approximately 15,000–20,000 events were acquired per sample. Data were calculated as the percentage of fluorescence of populations distributed in two-dimensional dot plots. Data were analyzed using FlowJow v10.0.6 software (Tree Star Inc., Ashland, OR, USA).

2.3. Statistical Analysis

The sample size was calculated using the following online tool: https://clincalc.com/Stats/SampleSize.aspx (accessed on 10 September 2024). The calculation was based on the media of total cholesterol (n = 14/group), rolling cells (n = 6/group), and carotid lesion area (n = 9/group) and was based on the apo E KO mice study. The C57BL/6 mice sample size was based on total cholesterol (n = 7/group) and 6 mice were used for bone marrow-derived macrophage. The analyses were performed using the GraphPad Prism 8.0 software (GraphPad Software, San Diego, CA, USA). Data were verified for the null hypothesis of Gaussian distribution using the Kolmogorov–Smirnov test. The Rout test was performed to identify outliers (that were excluded from the analyses). The statistical comparison of three or more groups was performed by one-way ANOVA, followed by Tukey's multiple comparisons post-test and Kruskal–Wallis test, with Dunns' multiple comparisons post-test for parametric and non-parametric data, respectively. When Cap groups were compared to their respective controls, the unpaired Student's t-test, and Mann–Whitney test were used for parametric and non-parametric data, respectively. The results were expressed as mean ± standard error (SE), with a significance level of 5%.

3. Results

3.1. Capsaicin Improves Weight, Reduces Visceral Fat, and Enhances Glycemia and Lipid Profile in ApoE KO Mice

There was no difference in caloric intake between the evaluated groups (Figure 1A). Despite this, weight gain (Figure 1B) and visceral fat percentage (Figure 1C) were reduced by approximately 50% in ApoE KO animals receiving Cap compared to their controls. Glycemia was higher in the ApoE KO group than in the WT group (Figure 1D), while the Cap groups presented intermediated glycemia levels (Figure 1D).

Regarding lipid profile, concentrations of triglycerides (Figure 1E), total cholesterol (Figure 1F), and non-HDL cholesterol (n-HDLc, Figure 1G) were reduced in ApoE + Cap mice without a reduction in HDL cholesterol (Figure 1H). These results suggest a beneficial effect of capsaicin intake on the lipid profile of the animals.

3.2. Capsaicin Reduces Inflammatory Markers in the Liver of ApoE KO Mice

As expected, ApoE KO mice exhibited heightened inflammatory markers compared to WT mice, except for IL-6 and IL-10 (Figure 2A–F). Supplementing ApoE KO mice with Cap reduced macrophage and neutrophil activity (measured by NAG and MPO enzyme activity, respectively) and TNF and IL1β concentrations to levels comparable to those in WT groups (Figure 2A–F). These findings suggest that Cap effectively regulates the basal inflammatory state in ApoE KO mice, bringing it closer to that of non-inflamed WT mice.

3.3. Capsaicin Treatment Reduces Atherosclerosis and Inflammation in ApoE KO Mice

Since C57Bl/6 mice would not develop atherosclerotic lesions in the short period used in this study, atherosclerosis development was only evaluated in ApoE KO groups by quantifying fatty streaks in the aorta and more advanced lesions in the carotid artery.

Capsaicin treatment significantly reduced the area affected by a fatty streak in the aorta, especially in the aortic arch (Figure 3A,B). Similarly, the carotid presented smaller lesions in the ApoE + Cap group compared to the ApoE KO group (Figure 3C,D). These findings suggest that Cap has an atheroprotective effect, as chronic intake effectively delays the development of both early-stage (fatty streak in the aorta) and more advanced (carotid lesions) atherosclerosis.

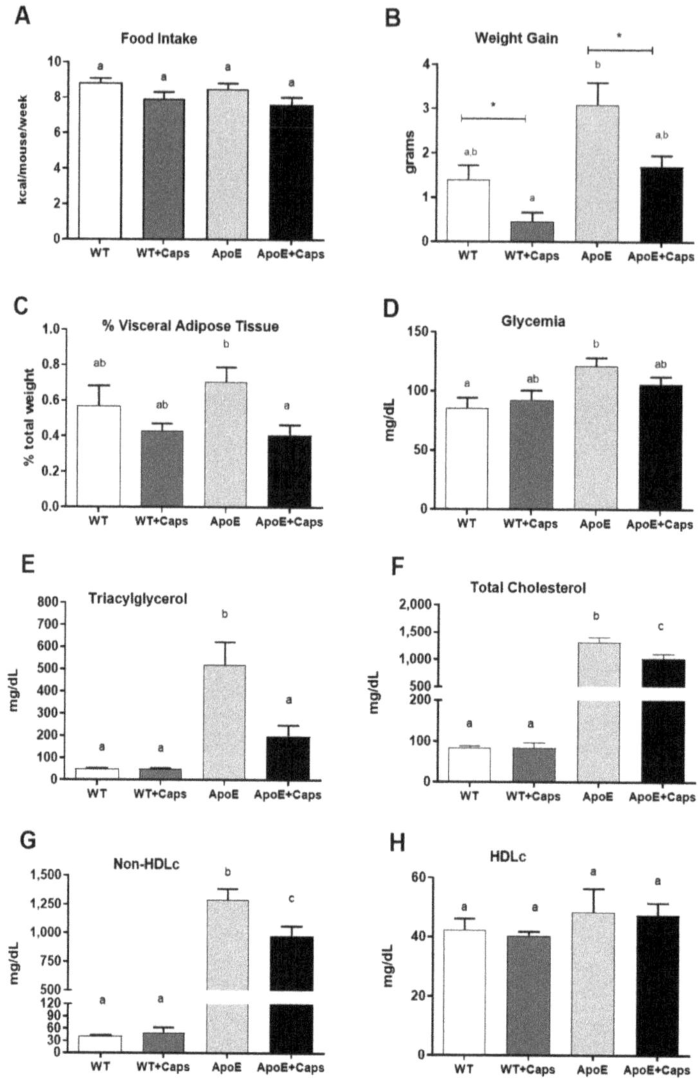

Figure 1. Effects of capsaicin on caloric intake, body composition, glycemia, and lipid profile in WT and ApoE-Deficient mice. Calorie intake (**A**), weight gain (**B**), fat percentage (**C**), glycemia (**D**), and lipid profile (**E–H**) of C57BL/6 and Apo E KO animals fed cholesterol-rich diet (AIN-93M + 0.75% cholesterol) without or with 0.015% capsaicin. Bars represent the mean, and vertical lines represent the standard error. Groups not sharing the same letter = statistically different. ($p < 0.05$). * T Student *t*-test compared with group without capsaicin. *N* mice = WT = 5, WT + CAP = 6, ApoE − KO = 11, ApoE + Cap = 10.

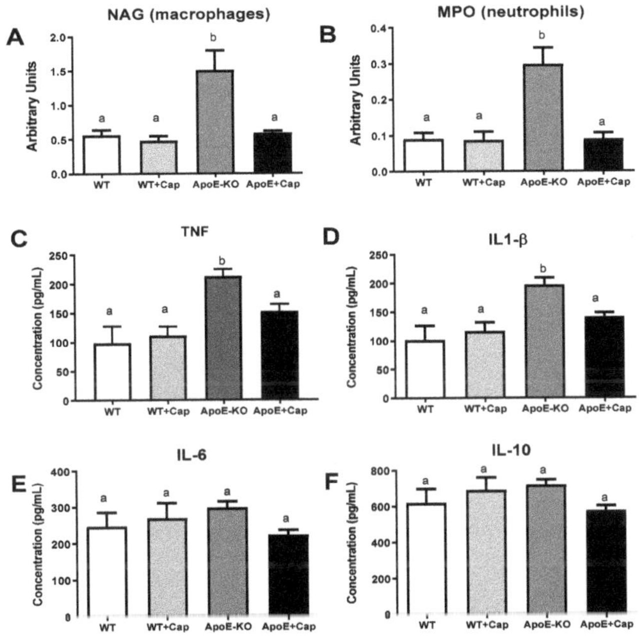

Figure 2. Modulation of Inflammatory Markers by Capsaicin in WT and ApoE KO Mice. Quantification of NAG (**A**), MPO (**B**), and the cytokines TNF (**C**), IL-1β (**D**), IL-6 (**E**), and IL-10 (**F**) in the liver tissue of wild-type animals (C57BL/6) and ApoE KO mice receiving control (AIN-93M + 0.075% cholesterol) or capsaicin-containing (AIN-93M + 0.075% cholesterol + 0.015% capsaicin) diets for 5 weeks. Data are presented as mean (bars) and standard error (vertical lines). Groups not sharing the same letter = statistically different ($p < 0.05$). N mice = WT = 5, WT + CAP = 6, ApoE − KO = 11, ApoE + Cap = 10, except for NAG and MPO n = 5–6 mice/group.

To investigate the role of macrophage-derived foam cells, we examined the presence of macrophages and their main scavenger receptor, CD36, in the lesion site. The results showed a reduced area of MOMA staining in lesions of Cap mice, indicating decreased monocyte/macrophage recruitment (Figure 3E,F). This was further confirmed by the lower density of CD36 in the same group (Figure 3G,H).

To determine if the observed improvements in the inflammatory state were systemic, we conducted an intravital microscopy experiment to observe the activation of circulating leukocytes in real-time. Investigating leukocyte rolling and adhesion via intravital microscopy is crucial, as these processes initiate inflammatory responses which are pivotal in atherosclerotic plaque development. The results revealed a significant reduction in the leukocyte rolling and adhesion in animals fed with Cap, suggesting a systemic anti-inflammatory effect of Cap (Figure 3I–L), Supplementary Videos S1 and S2. In summary, capsaicin treatment reduces atherosclerosis development, which is linked with decreased macrophage recruitment and CD36 expression in lesions, suggesting its role in inhibiting foam cell formation.

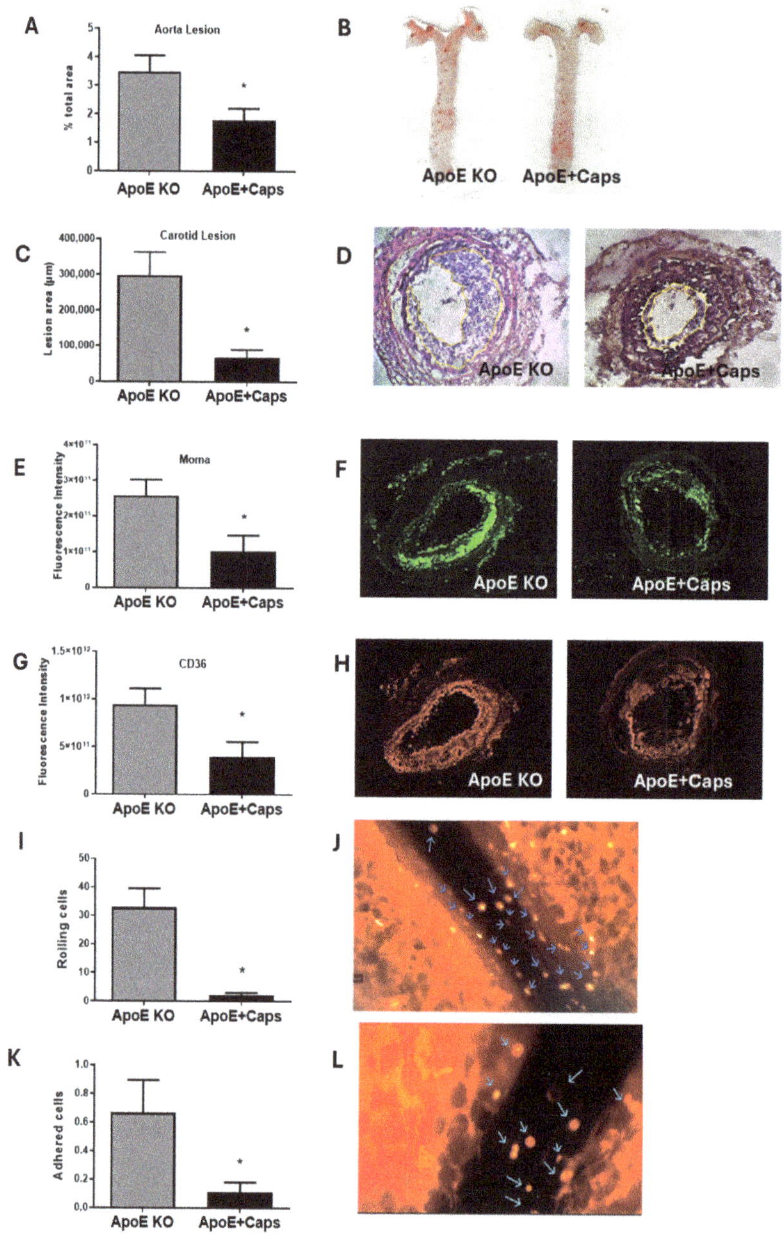

Figure 3. Effects of Capsaicin on Atherosclerosis Development and Inflammation (**A**,**B**) Percentage of the aorta affected by atherosclerotic lesions in ApoE KO mice after five weeks of ingesting a diet rich in cholesterol with or without Cap (0.015%) n = 8–9 mice/group (**C**,**D**)—Atherosclerotic lesion area in the obstructed carotid artery n = 7 mice/group. Fluoresce intensity of monocyte/macrophage (**E**,**F**) and CD36 (**G**,**H**) staining in the carotid artery (n = 7–10 mice/group). Rolling (**I**,**J**) and adhered (**K**,**L**) cells in the mesenteric plexus blood by intravital microscopy. Data are presented as mean (bars) and standard error (vertical lines). * Statistically different ($p < 0.05$). Blue arrows show rolling and adhering leukocytes. N mice = 6–8 mice/group.

3.4. Capsaicin Reduces Foam Cell Formation by Modulating Macrophage Cholesterol Influx and Efflux Pathways

After demonstrating the anti-atherosclerotic effects, we evaluated the influence of Cap on macrophage-derived foam cells by measuring the changes in oxLDL-loaded cells, expression of the influx-related receptors (CD36 and SRA), and the efflux-related transporter (ABCA1 and ABCG1). In BMDM cells pretreated with 1 or 5 μM Cap without any inhibitor, foam cells (oxLDL-Dil $^{+}$ cells) were reduced compared with non-treated cells (Figure 4A–F). This effect was accompanied by fewer cells expressing the SRA scavenger receptors (Figure 4B–G) without altering the number of CD36-expressing cells (Figure 4G,H). Regarding efflux transporters, Cap treatment increased the proportion of cells expressing ABCA1 in a 5 mM concentration (Figure 4D–I). Interestingly, the number of cells expressing ABCG1 decreased with both concentrations of Cap. (Figure 4E–J). These results suggest that Cap reduces foam cell formation by lowering cholesterol influx via SRA downregulation and increasing ABCA1-mediated efflux.

We investigated the influence of the natural Cap ligand, TRPV1, by treating cells with the TRPV1 inhibitor CZE. While TRPV1 inhibition increased foam cell formation, Cap's ability to reduce oxLDL uptake remained evident (Figure 4A). Confirming our previous data, foam cell increase was associated with increased SRA-expressing cells without effects on CD36-expressing cells (Figure 4B,C).

TRPV1 inhibition, however, did not affect ABCA1-expressing cells in control or 1 μM Cap-treated cells (Figure 4D), although a slight reduction of ABCA1 was seen with 5 μM treatment. Regarding the ABCG1 receptor, CZE treatment increased this transporter only in capsaicin-exposed cells, suggesting TRPV1 inhibits Cap's action on ABCG1 expression. Together, these data indicate that Cap's action in reducing cholesterol influx (via SRA) and ABCG1 is dependent on TRPV1, although the action on the ABCA1 transporter is independent of TRPV1.

Given that TRPV1 does not influence ABCA1, we investigated another target of capsaicin signaling, the PPARγ receptors. Our results showed that the inhibition of PPARγ, unlike what was seen with the TRPV1 inhibition, drastically reduced the foam cells in control and Cap-treated cells (Figure 4F) and was associated with the decreased cells expressing SRA and CD36 (Figure 4G,H). Nonetheless, Cap does not affect the CD36 receptors since there is no difference between Cap and the control groups. Regarding SRA, Cap has a small but significant effect at 5 μM after PPARγ inhibitor treatment.

When evaluating efflux transporters, PPARγ inhibition reduced the expression of ABCA1, abolishing the effect of the Cap (Figure 4I). However, the expression of ABCG1, although significantly reduced in CT cells, maintains the pattern seen in Cap cells without GW9662 treatment, showing a reduction in the number of cells expressing this transporter (Figure 4J). These results suggest that PPARγ promotes influx receptor expression and foam cell formation, while its inhibition drastically inhibits CD36 and SRA. Regarding efflux transporters, the increase of ABCA1 expression related to Cap treatment is dependent on PPARγ. Conversely, the ABCG1 expression seems to be favored by PPARγ activation, although the effect of Cap in reducing this transporter is independent of it.

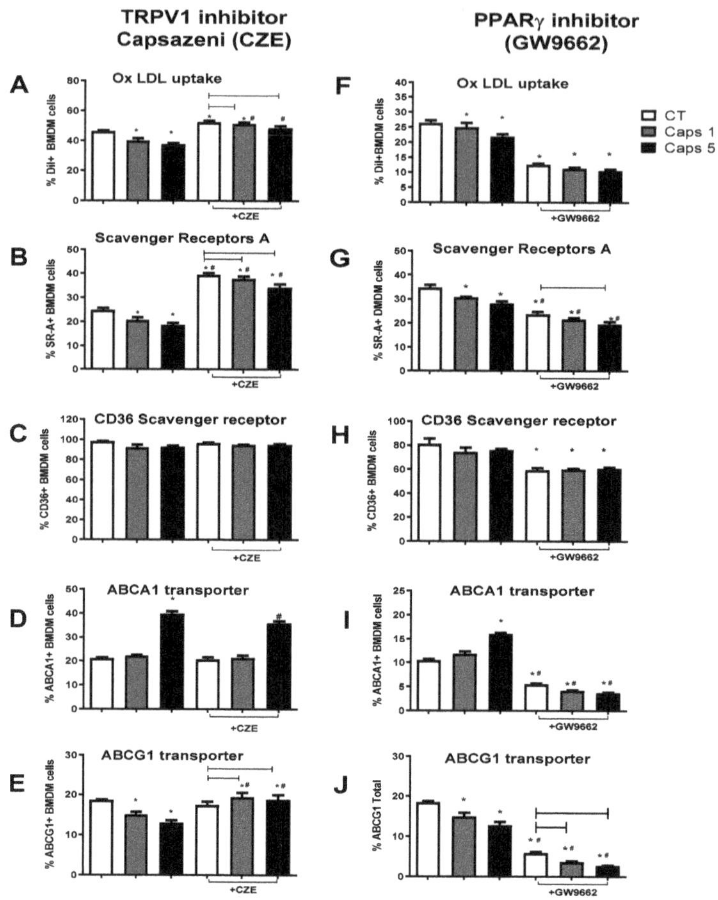

Figure 4. Cholesterol influx and efflux pathways in cultures treated without or with TRPV1 antagonist (CZE (**A–E**)) or PPARγ inhibitor (**F–J**). (**A**)—Total% of oxLDL-Dil positive populations treated or not with CZE; (**B**)—Total% of SRA-positive cells, treated or not with CZE; (**C**)—Total% of populations positive for CD36, treated or not with CZE; (**D**)—Total% of ABCA1-positive cells treated or not with CZE (**E**)—Total% of ABCG1-positive cells treated or not with CZE; (**F**)—Total% of oxLDL-Dil positive populations treated or not with GW9662; (**G**)—Total% of CD36-positive populations, treated or not with GW9662; (**H**)—Total% of SARS-positive cells, treated or not with GW9662; (**I**)—Total% of ABCA1-positive cells treated or not with GW9662; (**J**)—Total% of cells positive for ABCG1 treated or not with GW9662; Bars represent mean and vertical lines represent standard error (SE). Difference statistically significant ($p < 0.05$) is provided as (*) between each group (with or without inhibitors) and the control group (CT) without inhibitors; (—) between Caps groups treated with inhibitors and the CT group treated with inhibitors; (#) between groups treated with the inhibitor and the same group without the inhibitor.

4. Discussion

Our study demonstrated that capsaicin effectively reduces systemic inflammation, dyslipidemia, and atherosclerosis development in ApoE KO mice. The observed decrease in visceral adipose tissue, independent of food intake, aligns with existing literature on capsaicin's metabolic effects, enhanced lipolysis, and stimulation of browning [9,10,23,24]. Visceral fat is an important trigger of inflammation, and its reduction is crucial to improving the inflammatory state observed in both obesity and atherogenesis [9].

Hypercholesterolemia, particularly elevated levels of non-HDL cholesterol (atherogenic fraction) and, to a lesser extent, hypertriglyceridemia, are well-established risk factors for atherosclerosis. Our study, consistent with previous research, demonstrated an improvement in the lipid profile following capsaicin supplementation in several animal models and clinical trials, suggesting that capsaicin is a promising approach for reducing circulating levels of LDL-C in patients with metabolic syndrome [25].

Atherosclerosis involves the uptake of modified oxidized apo B-containing lipoproteins (non-HDL) by macrophages and smooth muscle cells (SMCs). This leads to foam cell formation via influx scavenger receptors such as SRA and CD36. Cholesterol efflux, regulated by ATP-binding cassette (ABC) transporters such as ABCA1 and ABCG1, is crucial for maintaining intracellular cholesterol homeostasis. ABCA1 facilitates the transfer of cholesterol and phospholipids to apoprotein A–I, forming nascent HDL, while ABCG1 promotes cholesterol efflux from macrophages to HDL [26]. Our study found that reducing non-HDLc while maintaining HDLc levels in the ApoE + Cap group was critical for delaying atherosclerosis progression in the aorta and reducing advanced lesions in the carotid artery.

The reduction of visceral adiposity, blood lipids, and atherosclerosis lesions, prompted us to investigate whether systemic inflammation was also diminished. Some inflammatory markers, including NAG, MPO, TNF, and IL-1β were significantly decreased. Notably, the reduction in MPO activity indicates not only an improvement in inflammation but also in oxidative status, as MPO activity involves reactive oxygen species (ROS) generation. MPO also contributes to chemical modifications, which increases foam cell formation [27].

High concentrations of TNF and IL-1β compromise the normal functioning of endothelial cells (EC), inducing oxidative stress, producing procoagulant factors, and impairing vasodilation, accelerating atherothrombosis [28]. Cap's reduction of hepatic inflammation could depend on TRPV1 activation because the reduced serum levels and hepatic expression of TNF and IL-1β in LPS-treated mice were not observed in TRPV1 knockout mice [29]. This effect was associated with the release of calcitonin gene-related peptide (CGRP), resulting from the activation of TRPV1.

To explore the systemic repercussions of capsaicin's anti-inflammatory effects, we used intravital microscopy to quantify leukocyte rolling and adhesion. The adherence of leukocytes to the vascular endothelium is a striking feature of the inflammatory process. Initial adhesive interactions between leukocytes and the endothelium involve tethering (capturing) and rolling. This initial weak interaction may become more robust by leukocyte activation, leading to stronger adhesion. These cells can then migrate into the interstitium through spaces between adjacent endothelial cells (ECs), initiated by various chemical mediators from the inflamed tissue [30]. Our study demonstrated that leukocyte rolling, and adhesion were reduced in animals fed with capsaicin, reinforcing the anti-inflammatory effects of this compound shown in the liver, aorta, and carotid. Schneider et al. [31] obtained similar results using intravital microscopy to explore the role of CGRP in acute pancreatitis in Wistar rats. The authors demonstrated that a capsaicin injection before pancreatitis induction could reduce tissue damage and 24-h mortality from pancreatitis by improving perfusion and reducing pancreatic inflammation.

Although our in vivo study highlighted the atheroprotective action of capsaicin, it also has some limitations. Firstly, the surgical carotid obstruction may not accurately replicate the natural development of atherosclerosis in humans, as it may not fully capture the complexity and variability of the disease process. Additionally, Apo E KO mice do not exhibit a lipoprotein profile identical to that of humans. This disparity can lead to significant differences in the progression and response to treatment of lipid-related diseases, such as atherosclerosis, which are closely linked to lipoprotein metabolism. Nonetheless, these limitations underscore the importance of complementing animal studies with additional research, using models or systems that more closely resemble human physiology or directly in human populations to ensure the relevance and applicability of the findings.

Capsaicin has been shown to reduce the inflammatory response by regulating intracellular lipid overload [20,32,33]. However, there is no consensus on the exact mechanisms mediating this process. Some studies suggest that Cap minimizes cholesterol load and inflammation in foam cells independently of TRPV1 [20,32,33], potentially by regulating cholesterol efflux via LXR-α and PPARγ [25,34]. In contrast, other studies demonstrate that TRPV1 signaling is essential for Cap to prevent foam cell formation [29].

Our experiments revealed that Cap pre-treatment reduces LDL-loaded foam cells by modulating the expression of influx and efflux receptors through pathways involving TRPV1 and PPARγ. Cap significantly reduced the expression of SRA, dependent on the TRPV1 activation. Inhibition or deficiency of TRPV1 abolished this reduction, while PPARγ inhibition decreased SRA-expressing cells. This PPAR-mediated action was previously observed in SMC-derived foam cells, where PPARγ expression induces CD36 expression and subsequent lipid accumulation [35,36]. Our results in BMDMs align with these findings, showing reduced CD36 and SRA expression following PPARγ inhibition. Although we did not measure the expression of PPARγ target genes to confirm the inhibitory effect of GW9662 in our experimental model, our study demonstrated that this antagonist influenced the expression of both efflux and influx receptors in BMDM cells, with significant alterations observed in both control and Caps-treated cells. Supporting our results, Martin-Fuentes et al. [37] showed that CD36 expression in macrophages derived from human monocytes incubated with ox-LDL is mainly regulated by pro-inflammatory cytokines, while SR-A expression correlates with PPARγ and NF-kB. Thus, PPARγ activation by capsaicin in the absence of functional TRPV1 increases in SRA-expressing foam cells.

In the presence of TRPV1, as observed in BMDMs without antagonism, Cap reduced the foam cell population modestly (approximately 13%) but significantly, suggesting that TRPV1 activation overrides the PPARγ effect of increasing SRA. Additionally, treating cells with PPARγ inhibitors highlights the role of TRPV1 activation in reducing SRA and CD36 expression, as neither Cap nor oxLDL alone effectively induced the expression of influx receptors, leading to a significant reduction in foam cell population.

Our study is innovative as it covers not only the risk factors for atherosclerosis but also the characterization of biomarkers for the development of both early and advanced lesions. It highlights the importance of antioxidants and, especially, the anti-inflammatory action of capsaicin in this process. The study also proposes a mechanism related to the formation and modulation of foam cells in macrophages. Therefore, our results make significant contributions and pave the way for clinical studies.

5. Conclusions

In conclusion, capsaicin demonstrates significant potential in reducing atherosclerosis progression by modulating cholesterol metabolism and inflammation while inhibiting foam cell formation. Also, our data suggest that Cap effectively reduces oxLDL-loaded foam cells by downregulating the scavenger receptor SRA and increasing the efflux transporter ABCA1. Importantly, these effects are partially mediated by TRPV1 and independent of PPARγ activation. In the absence of functional TRPV1, Cap exerts a more modest effect on foam cell reduction. PPARγ activation by Cap in vitro reduces cholesterol efflux and increases influx scavenger receptors. Mechanistic insights into capsaicin's actions involving TRPV1 and PPARγ pathways provide further rationale for exploring its clinical applications in managing atherosclerosis and related complications.

Supplementary Materials: The following supporting information can be downloaded at: https://www.mdpi.com/article/10.3390/nu16183167/s1, Supplementary Video S1, and Supplementary Video S2.

Author Contributions: Conceptualization, J.I.A.-L.; methodology, D.L.Á., W.F.-B., J.L.S., E.A.S., G.C., L.S.A.C., E.C.A. and P.C.L.L., formal analysis, D.L.Á., W.F.-B., E.C.A. and J.I.A.-L.; investigation, D.L.Á.; writing, D.L.Á., J.I.A.-L. and W.F.-B. All authors have read and agreed to the published version of the manuscript.

Funding: The Fundação Coordenação de Aperfeiçoamento de Pessoal de Nível Superior (CAPES) #001 and the Conselho Nacional de Desenvolvimento Científico e Tecnológico (CNPq) #310571/2020-0 financially supported this study.

Institutional Review Board Statement: The animal study protocol was approved by the Ethics Committee of Animal Experimentation—UFMG (# 232/2016, 20 September 2016).

Informed Consent Statement: Not applicable.

Data Availability Statement: The datasets analyzed during the current study are available from the corresponding author upon reasonable request.

Acknowledgments: We acknowledge Maria Helena Alves Oliveira for the animal care.

Conflicts of Interest: The authors declare no conflicts of interest.

References

1. Chanda, S.; Bashir, M.; Babbar, S.; Koganti, A.; Bley, K. In vitro hepatic and skin metabolism of capsaicin. *Drug Metab. Dispos.* **2008**, *36*, 670–675. (In English) [CrossRef] [PubMed]
2. TMaximiano, T.K.E.; Carneiro, J.A.; Fattori, V.; Verri, W.A. TRPV1: Receptor structure, activation, modulation and role in neuro-immune interactions and pain. *Cell Calcium* **2024**, *119*, 102870. (In English) [CrossRef] [PubMed]
3. Silva, J.L.; Santos, E.A.; Alvarez-Leite, J.I. Are We Ready to Recommend Capsaicin for Disorders Other Than Neuropathic Pain? *Nutrients* **2023**, *15*, 4469. (In English) [CrossRef]
4. Nawaka, N.; Wanmasae, S.; Makarasen, A.; Dechtrirat, D.; Techasakul, S.; Jeenduang, N. Allicin and Capsaicin Ameliorated Hypercholesterolemia by Upregulating LDLR and Downregulating PCSK9 Expression in HepG2 Cells. *Int. J. Mol. Sci.* **2022**, *23*, 14299. (In English) [CrossRef]
5. Huang, C.-J.; Pu, C. M.; Su, S. Y.; Lo, S.-L.; Lee, C.H.; Yen, Y.-H. Improvement of wound healing by capsaicin through suppression of the inflammatory response and amelioration of the repair process. *Mol. Med. Rep.* **2023**, *28*, 155. (In English) [CrossRef]
6. Irving, G.A.; Backonja, M.; Rauck, R.; Webster, L.R.; Tobias, J.K.; Vanhove, G.F. NGX-4010, a capsaicin 8% dermal patch, administered alone or in combination with systemic neuropathic pain medications, reduces pain in patients with postherpetic neuralgia. *Clin. J. Pain* **2012**, *28*, 101–107. (In English) [CrossRef] [PubMed]
7. Thongin, S.; Den-Udom, T.; Uppakara, K.; Sriwantana, T.; Sibmooh, N.; Laolob, T.; Boonthip, C.; Wichai, U.; Muta, K.; Ketsawatsomkron, P. Beneficial effects of capsaicin and dihydrocapsaicin on endothelial inflammation, nitric oxide production and antioxidant activity. *Biomed. Pharmacother.* **2022**, *154*, 113521. (In English) [CrossRef] [PubMed]
8. Zhang, W.; Zhang, Y.; Fan, J.; Feng, Z.; Song, X. Pharmacological activity of capsaicin: Mechanisms and controversies (Review). *Mol. Med. Rep.* **2024**, *29*, 38. (In English) [CrossRef]
9. Kim, H.J. Capsaicin supplementation prevents western diet-induced hyperleptinemia by reducing endoplasmic reticulum stress in apolipoprotein E-deficient mice. *Food Nutr. Res.* **2023**, *67*. (In English) [CrossRef]
10. Kang, J.-H.; Tsuyoshi, G.; Le Ngoc, H.; Kim, H.-M.; Tu, T.H.; Noh, H.-J.; Kim, C.-S.; Choe, S.-Y.; Kawada, T.; Yoo, H.; et al. Dietary capsaicin attenuates metabolic dysregulation in genetically obese diabetic mice. *J. Med. Food* **2011**, *14*, 310–315. (In English) [CrossRef]
11. Nam, D.; Ni, C.-W.; Rezvan, A.; Suo, J.; Budzyn, K.; Llanos, A.; Harrison, D.G.; Giddens, D.P.; Jo, H. A model of disturbed flow-induced atherosclerosis in mouse carotid artery by partial ligation and a simple method of RNA isolation from carotid endothelium. *J. Vis. Exp.* **2010**, *40*, e1861. (In English) [CrossRef]
12. Aguilar, E.; Leonel, A.; Teixeira, L.; Silva, A.; Silva, J.; Pelaez, J.; Capettini, L.; Lemos, V.; Santos, R.; Alvarez-Leite, J. Butyrate impairs atherogenesis by reducing plaque inflammation and vulnerability and decreasing NFκB activation. *Nutr. Metab. Cardiovasc. Dis.* **2014**, *24*, 606–613. (In English) [CrossRef] [PubMed]
13. Vieira, E.L.; Leonel, A.J.; Sad, A.P.; Beltrão, N.R.; Costa, T.F.; Ferreira, T.M.; Gomes-Santos, A.C.; Faria, A.M.; Peluzio, M.C.; Cara, D.C.; et al. Oral administration of sodium butyrate attenuates inflammation and mucosal lesion in experimental acute ulcerative colitis. *J. Nutr. Biochem.* **2012**, *23*, 430–436. (In English) [CrossRef]
14. Teixeira, L.G.; Leonel, A.J.; Aguilar, E.C.; Batista, N.V.; Alves, A.C.; Coimbra, C.C.; Ferreira, A.V.; De Faria, A.M.C.; Cara, D.C.; Alvarez Leite, J.I. The combination of high-fat diet-induced obesity and chronic ulcerative colitis reciprocally exacerbates adipose tissue and colon inflammation. *Lipids Health Dis.* **2011**, *10*, 204. (In English) [CrossRef] [PubMed]
15. Chung, B.H.; Segrest, J.P.; Ray, M.J.; Brunzell, J.D.; Hokanson, J.E.; Krauss, R.M.; Beaudrie, K.; Cone, J.T. Single vertical spin density gradient ultracentrifugation. *Methods Enzymol.* **1986**, *128*, 181–209. (In English) [CrossRef]
16. Lowry, O.H.; Rosebrough, N.J.; Farr, A.L.; Randall, R.J. Protein measurement with the Folin phenol reagent. *J. Biol. Chem.* **1951**, *193*, 265–275. (In English) [CrossRef]
17. Stephan, Z.F.; Yurachek, E.C. Rapid fluorometric assay of LDL receptor activity by DiI-labeled LDL. *J. Lipid Res.* **1993**, *34*, 325–330. (In English) [CrossRef]

18. Fernandes-Braga, W.; Aguilar, E.C.; Navia-Pelaez, J.M.; Ávila, D.L.; Rezende, L.; Andrade, L.d.O.; Miranda, S.E.M.; de Barros A.L.B.; Capettini, L.d.S.A.; Alvarez-Leite, J.I. The atheroprotective role of fucoidan involves the reduction of foam cell formation by altering cholesterol flux-associated factors in macrophages. *Biochem. Biophys. Res. Commun.* **2003**, *650*, 21–29. (In English [CrossRef]
19. Chen, C.; Lee, S.T.; Wu, W.T.; Fu, W.; Ho, F.; Lin, W.W. Signal transduction for inhibition of inducible nitric oxide synthase and cyclooxygenase-2 induction by capsaicin and related analogs in macrophages. *Br. J. Pharmacol.* **2003**, *140*, 1077–1087. (In English [CrossRef]
20. Zhao, J.-F.; Ching, L.-C.; Kou, Y.R.; Lin, S.-J.; Wei, J.; Shyue, S.-K.; Lee, T.-S. Activation of TRPV1 prevents OxLDL-induced lipid accumulation and TNF-α-induced inflammation in macrophages: Role of liver X receptor α. *Mediat. Inflamm.* **2013**, *2013*, 925171 (In English) [CrossRef]
21. Min, K.-W.; Zhang, X.; Imchen, T.; Baek, S.J. A peroxisome proliferator-activated receptor ligand MCC-555 imparts anti proliferative response in pancreatic cancer cells by PPARgamma-independent up-regulation of KLF4. *Toxicol. Appl. Pharmacol* **2012**, *263*, 225–232. (In English) [CrossRef] [PubMed]
22. Shiota, A.; Shimabukuro, M.; Fukuda, D.; Soeki, T.; Sato, H.; Uematsu, E.; Hirata, Y.; Kurobe, H.; Maeda, N.; Sakaue, H.; et al Telmisartan ameliorates insulin sensitivity by activating the AMPK/SIRT1 pathway in skeletal muscle of obese db/db mice *Cardiovasc. Diabetol.* **2012**, *11*, 139. (In English) [CrossRef] [PubMed]
23. Li, L.; Chen, J.; Ni, Y.; Feng, X.; Zhao, Z.; Wang, P.; Sun, J.; Yu, H.; Yan, Z.; Liu, D.; et al. TRPV1 activation prevents nonalcoholic fatty liver through UCP2 upregulation in mice. *Pflug. Arch.* **2012**, *463*, 727–732. (In English) [CrossRef]
24. Ohyama, K.; Nogusa, Y.; Suzuki, K.; Shinoda, K.; Kajimura, S.; Bannai, M. A combination of exercise and capsinoid supplementation additively suppresses diet-induced obesity by increasing energy expenditure in mice. *Am. J. Physiol. Endocrinol. Metab.* **2013** *308*, E315–E323. (In English) [CrossRef] [PubMed]
25. Hu, Y.-W.; Ma, X.; Huang, J.-L.; Mao, X.-R.; Yang, J.-Y.; Zhao, J.-Y.; Li, S.-F.; Qiu, Y.-R.; Yang, J.; Zheng, L.; et al. Dihydrocapsaicin Attenuates Plaque Formation through a PPARγ/LXRα Pathway in apoE(−/−) Mice Fed a High-Fat/High-Cholesterol Diet *PLoS ONE* **2013**, *8*, e66876. (In English) [CrossRef] [PubMed]
26. Zheng, Y.; Shao, M.; Zheng, Y.; Sun, W.; Qin, S.; Sun, Z.; Zhu, L.; Guan, Y.; Wang, Q.; Wang, Y.; et al. PPARs in atherosclerosis: The spatial and temporal features from mechanism to druggable targets. *J. Adv. Res.* **2024**, *29*. (In English) [CrossRef]
27. Khan, A.A.; Alsahli, M.A.; Rahmani, A.H. Myeloperoxidase as an Active Disease Biomarker: Recent Biochemical and Pathological Perspectives. *Med. Sci.* **2018**, *6*, 33. (In English) [CrossRef]
28. González, L.; Rivera, K.; Andia, M.E.; Rodriguez, G.M. The IL-1 Family and Its Role in Atherosclerosis. *Int. J. Mol. Sci.* **2022**, *24*, 17. (In English) [CrossRef]
29. Ma, L.; Zhong, J.; Zhao, Z.; Luo, Z.; Ma, S.; Sun, J.; He, H.; Zhu, T.; Liu, D.; Zhu, Z.; et al. Activation of TRPV1 reduces vascular lipid accumulation and attenuates atherosclerosis. *Cardiovasc. Res.* **2011**, *92*, 504–513. (In English) [CrossRef]
30. McEver, R.P.; Zhu, C. Rolling cell adhesion. *Annu. Rev. Cell Dev. Biol.* **2010**, *26*, 363–396. (In English) [CrossRef]
31. Schneider, L.; Hackert, T.; Heck, M.; Hartwig, W.; Fritz, S.; Strobel, O.; Gebhard, M.-M.; Werner, J. Capsaicin reduces tissue damage in experimental acute pancreatitis. *Pancreas* **2009**, *38*, 676–680. (In English) [CrossRef] [PubMed]
32. Kim, C.-S.; Kawada, T.; Kim, B.-S.; Han, I.-S.; Choe, S.-Y.; Kurata, T.; Yu, R. Capsaicin exhibits anti-inflammatory property by inhibiting IkB-a degradation in LPS-stimulated peritoneal macrophages. *Cell Signal* **2003**, *15*, 299–306. (In English) [CrossRef] [PubMed]
33. Park, Y.M.; Febbraio, M.; Silverstein, R.L. CD36 modulates migration of mouse and human macrophages in response to oxidized LDL and may contribute to macrophage trapping in the arterial intima. *J. Clin. Investig.* **2009**, *119*, 136–145. (In English) [CrossRef] [PubMed]
34. Tang, J.; Luo, K.; Li, Y.; Chen, Q.; Tang, D.; Wang, D.; Xiao, J. Capsaicin attenuates LPS-induced inflammatory cytokine production by upregulation of LXRalpha. *Int. Immunopharmacol.* **2015**, *28*, 264–269. (In English) [CrossRef] [PubMed]
35. Lim, H.-J.; Lee, S.; Lee, K.-S.; Park, J.-H.; Jang, Y.; Lee, E.J.; Park, H.-Y. PPARgamma activation induces CD36 expression and stimulates foam cell like changes in rVSMCs. *Prostaglandins Other Lipid Mediat.* **2006**, *80*, 165–174. (In English) [CrossRef]
36. Lazar, M.A. Progress in cardiovascular biology: PPAR for the course. *Nat. Med.* **2001**, *7*, 23–24. (In English) [CrossRef]
37. Martín-Fuentes, P.; Civeira, F.; Recalde, D.; García-Otín, A.L.; Jarauta, E.; Marzo, I.; Cenarro, A. Individual variation of scavenger receptor expression in human macrophages with oxidized low-density lipoprotein is associated with a differential inflammatory response. *J. Immunol.* **2007**, *179*, 3242–3248. (In English) [CrossRef]

nutrients

MDPI

Article

Herbal Extracts Mixed with Essential Oils: A Network Approach for Gastric and Intestinal Motility Disorders

Roberta Budriesi [1,*,†], Ivan Corazza [2,†], Simone Roncioni [3], Roberta Scanferlato [3], Dalila De Luca [3], Carla Marzetti [3], Roberto Gotti [4,*], Nicola Rizzardi [5], Christian Bergamini [5], Matteo Micucci [6], Davide Roncarati [7] and Laura Beatrice Mattioli [1]

1 Food Chemistry and Nutraceutical Laboratory, Department of Pharmacy and Biotechnology (FaBiT), Alma Mater Studiorum-University of Bologna, Via Belmeloro 6, 40126 Bologna, Italy; laurabeatrice.mattioli@unibo.it
2 Department of Medical and Surgical Sciences (DIMEC), Alma Mater Studiorum-University of Bologna, 40138 Bologna, Italy; ivan.corazza@unibo.it
3 Valsambro S.r.l., 40121 Bologna, Italy; simone.roncioni@gmail.com (S.R.); r.scanferlato@hotmail.com (R.S.); dalila.deluca@valsambro.it (D.D.L.); carla.marzetti@valsambro.it (C.M.)
4 Department of Pharmacy and Biotechnology (FaBiT), University of Bologna, Via Belmeloro 6, 40126 Bologna, Italy
5 Department of Pharmacy and Biotechnology (FaBiT), University of Bologna, Via Irnerio 48, 40126 Bologna, Italy; nicola.rizzardi2@unibo.it (N.R.); christian.bergamini2@unibo.it (C.B.)
6 Department of Biomolecular Sciences, University of Urbino "Carlo Bo", 61029 Urbino, Italy; matteo.micucci@uniurb.it
7 Department of Pharmacy and Biotechnology (FaBiT), University of Bologna, Via Selmi 3, 40126 Bologna, Italy; davide.roncarati@unibo.it
* Correspondence: roberta.budriesi@unibo.it (R.B.), roberto.gotti@unibo.it (R.G.)
† These authors contributed equally to this work.

Abstract: Background: Three herbal extracts (*Asparagus racemosus* Willd., *Tabebuia avellanedae* Lorentz, and *Glycyrrhiza glabra* L.) were mixed with three essential oils (*Foeniculum vulgare* Mill., *Mentha piperita* L., and *Pimpinella anisum* L.) to formulate a product (HEMEO) whose active compounds include saponins and steroids in *Asparagus racemosus*, known for their anti-inflammatory properties; glycyrrhizin and flavonoids in *Glycyrrhiza glabra*, which exhibit gastroprotective and antispasmodic effects; menthol in *Mentha piperita*, contributing with antispasmodic and antimicrobial properties; and anethole and polyphenols in *Pimpinella anisum*, which modulate intestinal motility and offer antimicrobial activity. Objective: HEMEO was formulated for applications in intestinal motility disorders. Methods: HEMEO was evaluated for spontaneous and induced motility effects in isolated guinea pig ileum, colon, and stomach. Ex vivo experiments were conducted using LabChart software v7.0, and the product's antibacterial action against *Helicobacter pylori* and its antioxidant effects were assessed through disc diffusion and FRAP assays. The presence of the volatile compounds in the formulation was confirmed by GC-MS analysis; the TPC of HEMEO, determined using the Folin–Ciocalteu method, was 9.925 ± 0.42 mg GAE/g. Conclusions: HEMEO showed a phenolic content correlated with its antioxidant potential and in addition inhibited *H. pylori* growth and demonstrated notable antioxidant properties, suggesting its role as a supportive agent in digestive processes and in managing motility disorders.

Keywords: *Asparagus racemosus* Willd.; *Tabebuia avellanedae* Lorentz; *Glycyrrhiza glabra* L.; *Helicobacter pylori*; tissues contractility; antioxidant activity; essential oils

1. Introduction

The gastrointestinal (GI) tract performs various functions, including digestion and absorption [1]. Motility, the muscular activity of the GI tract, plays a key role in the digestive process across different parts of the intestinal tract [2,3]. Normal motility involves a sequence of muscular contractions from top to bottom [4]. When motility is abnormal, with contractions that are too rapid, slow, or disorganized, pain can arise due to brain–gut communication [5]. Central nervous system processing in visceral hypersensitivity causes functional dysfunctions and pain [6,7]. "Intestinal motility disorders" are characterized by abnormal intestinal contractions (spasms and paralysis), where the gut loses its ability to coordinate motor function due to endogenous or exogenous causes or infection. With its muscular solid walls, the stomach holds food and mixes it with acid and enzymes into a liquid paste, playing a crucial role in the digestive process. However, food or drugs can compromise the delicate balance that regulates this organ's functionality [8]. Functional minor and colonic disorders involve middle or lower GI tract symptoms, impacting the absorption of nutrients, vitamins (small intestine), water, and electrolytes (colon). Functional motility disorders include inflammatory bowel syndrome (IBS), functional bloating, functional constipation, functional diarrhea, and unspecified functional bowel disorders. The human gut microbiome, a heterogeneous microbial system, regulates intestinal physiology and pathology. Disruption of this microbial equilibrium can break the epithelial barrier, causing hypersensitivity and abnormalities in gut motility [9].

This paper focuses on a pathogenic bacterium, *Helicobacter pylori* (*H. pylori*), which infects and causes inflammation and ulcers in the stomach or small intestine. *H. pylori* is very common, affecting about two-thirds of the world's population [10]. Many studies demonstrate an association between H. pylori and disorders outside of the stomach [11], demonstrating how the infection also influences pathologies of the extragastric intestinal tract [12]. In particular, *H. pylori* infection appears to be able to modify the intestinal microbiota by altering the release of local chemical mediators that influence the host's immune response [13].

Herbal mixtures are widely used in traditional Chinese medicine to target various aspects of pathologies [14–18]. In this context, a multitarget approach to addressing different mechanisms associated with the same pathology is of great importance for effective symptom management. It is well-established that disorders related to impaired motility often require various drugs acting on multiple therapeutic targets [19]. The "network target" approach we propose is based on a mixture of organic compounds within the extracts, capable of interacting with multiple targets [20]. This strategy involves evaluating the activity of the extracts on individual targets associated with the pathology. Furthermore, combining different herbal extracts aims to broaden the range of targets the therapy addresses while minimizing effects on targets unrelated to the pathological network. HEMEO, the focus of this study, is a multi-component herbal formula designed to address GI motility disorders by leveraging the active compounds in each of its herbal and essential oil constituents. Each plant extract contributes specific bioactive compounds with targeted effects. The herbal mixture consists of extracts from *Asparagus racemosus* Willd. Oberm (racemose asparagus), *Tabebuia avellanedae* Lorentz ex Griseb (lapacho), and *Glycyrrhiza glabra* L. (licorice). *Asparagus racemosus* contains saponins and steroidal compounds, primarily shatavarins, which exhibit anti-inflammatory and antiulcerogenic impact, making this herb useful for managing gastric discomfort and supporting digestive health [21–24]. Studies by Bhatnagar et al. demonstrate that *Asparagus racemosus* reduces gastric emptying time [25], a phenomenon linked to duodenal ulcer and gastric HCl release [26], and presents significant antidiarrheal action by inhibiting intestinal motility [27]. *Tabebuia avellanedae,* known as "lapacho", has gastroprotective action [28] and is used in traditional medicine for treating ulcers and infections [29]. *Glycyrrhiza glabra* roots are rich in glycyrrhizin (18 β-glycyrrhetinic acid), an essential compound for preventing gastroduodenal ulcers and reducing pain. This gastroprotective action is complemented by flavonoids, which collectively contribute to licorice's role in soothing the GI tract. However, licorice use has been associated with side effects, particularly hypertension, due to glycyrrhizin's influence on sodium retention and potassium loss [30]. The gastrointestinal effects are further enhanced by isoliquiritigenin, a bioactive flavonoid that induces spasmolytic effects by blocking calcium channels, helping to alleviate smooth muscle spasms and thus improving GI comfort [31]. The distinctive feature of the selected herbal formulation lies in the presence of essential oils. Essential oils, in general, inhibit critical steps of bacterial infections, including biofilm formation and toxin production, which are pivotal for maintaining intestinal homeostasis [32]. Moreover, the intestinal microbiota plays a crucial role in maintaining colon homeostasis, mitigating many adverse effects caused by chemical compounds in foods and during infections. In this context, the selective activity of essential oils against pathogenic bacterial populations presents a particularly compelling area of interest [33].

Three essential oils from *Foeniculum Vulgare* Mill. (fennel), *Mentha piperita* L. (peppermint), and *Pimpinella Anisum* L. (anise) complement the herbal extract. Fennel is commonly used in traditional medicine for various digestive disorders [34] and is praised for its antimicrobial and antifungal action [35]. Its essential oil regulates intestinal motility and is used for gastrointestinal atony and stomach heaviness [36–38]. Anethole, found mainly in fennel seeds, has anti-cancer properties [39]. Peppermint, rich in menthol, this provides as an essential oil antispasmodic and antimicrobial properties. Menthol interacts with calcium channels and provides soothing effects on intestinal muscle, making it beneficial in managing spasms related to GI disturbances [40,41]. Both fennel and peppermint have antispasmodic actions on smooth muscles and influence gastric and salivary secretion. Anise essential oil contains anethole and polyphenols, which modulate GI motility and offer antimicrobial effects that may help balance intestinal flora. Anise is widely used to alleviate bloating and discomfort associated with digestive issues [38,42].

All these extracts and essential oils act on the gastrointestinal tract and modulate targets linked to GI functional disorders. Therapies based on the "one drug, one target, one disease" approach have gradually shifted towards adopting multiple active component treatment strategies [43]. Our study analyzed the synergistic effect of active ingredients on a network of gastrointestinal targets. Therefore, it is a multitarget-get-multicomponent approach, which allows for the pathology to be treated globally, considering "more drugs and more targets".

This study evaluated the effect of HEMEO on the basal and induced contractility of guinea pigs' stomach, ileum, and colon, as well as its effect on *H. pylori* and its antioxidant properties. The cardiovascular impact of HEMEO was also studied to provide a comprehensive overview of this herbal mixture's off-target activity. Figure 1 shows the experimental design.

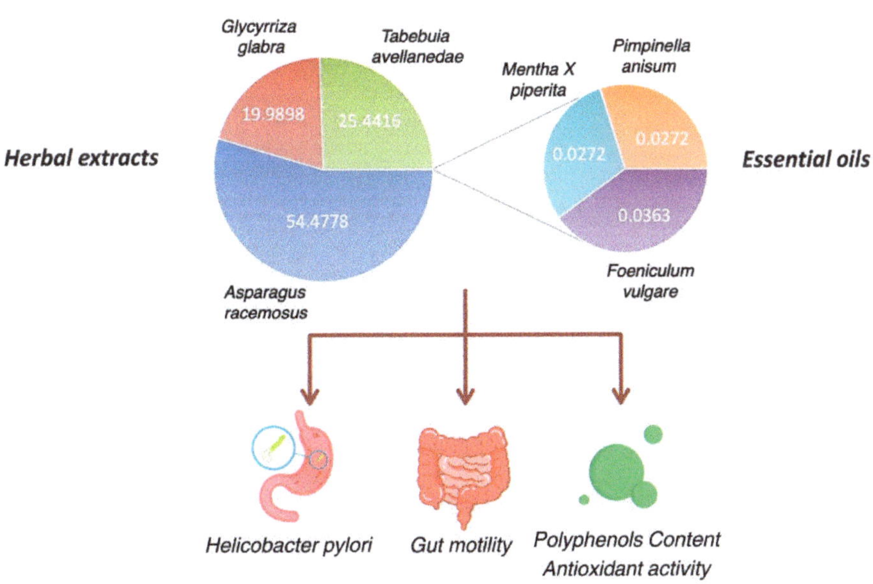

Figure 1. Overview of experimental design of HEMEO.

2. Materials and Methods

2.1. HEMEO Chemical Composition

The composition of the herbal extracts mixed with essential oils, kindly provided by Homeo Sapiens, Cesena (FC), Italy, is as follows: *Asparagus racemosus* Willd. Oberm 300 mg (54.4778%); *Tabebuia avellanedae* Lorentz ex Griseb 140 mg (25.4416%), containing 3% naphthoquinones as lapachol equivalent to 4.2 mg; *Glycyrrhiza glabra* L. 110 mg (19.9898%), containing triterpenic saponins with 19% glycyrrhizic acid; *Foeniculum vulgare* Mill. essential oil 0.200 mg (0.0363%); *Mentha X piperita* L. essential oil 0.150 mg (0.0272%); *Pimpinella anisum* L. essential oil 0.150 mg (0.0272%) (Figure 2).

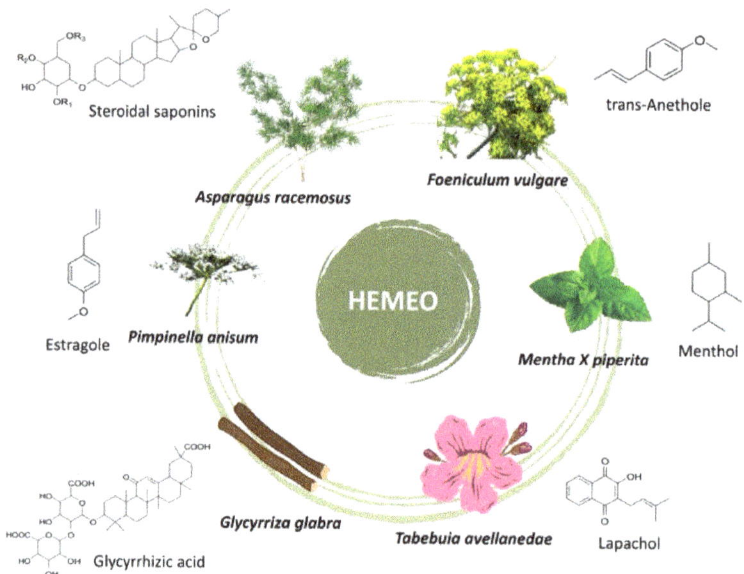

Figure 2. Plants pictures and chemical structure of key compounds found in the plant extracts and essential oils.

2.1.1. Identification of Essential Oils Components

GC-MS instrumentation and conditions. The chromatographic experiments to identify the terpenes associated with the essential oils of HEMEO were carried out on a GC-MS Gas Chromatograph by Agilent Technologies (Santa Clara, CA, USA), model 8890 combined with the Mass detector (MS) Agilent model 5977B. The chromatographic conditions were as follows: the capillary column was an Rtx® 5 MS column (30 m × 0.25 mm ID, 0.25 μm) Crossbond® (5% phenyl–95% dimethylpolysiloxane) by (Restek, Cernusco sul Naviglio, Milano, Italy); the carrier gas was helium at the flow rate of 1 mL/min; the temperature program was initial temperature of 40 °C (hold time: 5 min), followed by a ramp at 7 °C/min to 230 °C (hold time: 5 min). The injector base, transfer line, and ionization source temperatures were 280, 250, and 200 °C, respectively. The Gas Chromatograph (GC) was operated in split mode using a split ratio of 1:50. The electron ionization (EI at 70 eV) was used, and the mass spectra were recorded in full scan mode (50–650 amu) to collect the total ion current (TIC) chromatograms. The terpenes were identified by comparing retention time and mass spectrum with authentic standards as reference. The identity confirmation was carried out by comparing the mass spectra of the analytes with those of the NIST (National Institute of Standards and Technology, Gaithersburg, MD, USA) library version 2.4 (2020).

Sample preparation for GC-MS analysis. The samples to be subjected to GC-MS analysis were prepared by extracting an amount of 1 mg of the HEMEO powder using dichloromethane (1 mL) under ultrasonication using an ultrasonic bath for 5 min. The suspension was filtered (0.45 μm) before injecting into the gas chromatograph.

2.1.2. Determination of Total Phenolic Content (TPC)

The total phenolic content (TPC) in HEMEO was determined using a slightly modified Folin–Ciocalteu method [44,45]. A calibration curve was established using a series of gallic acid standards (50–500 μg/mL of gallic acid solution in water). For each standard and sample, 50 μL was combined with 250 μL of Folin–Ciocalteu reagent and allowed to react for 5 min. Subsequently, 1 mL of 20% Na_2CO_3 was added, and the mixture was diluted with demineralized water to a final volume of 5 mL. The solutions were then incubated at room temperature for 30 min, and absorbance was measured at 760 nm using a spectrophotometer (Jasco V-730, Jasco Europe SrL, Cremella, Italy). The TPC of the samples was expressed as Gallic Acid Equivalents (GAEs) in mg/g, calculated from the calibration curve.

2.2. *Ex Vivo Studies*

2.2.1. Animals

Male guinea pigs (200–400 g) obtained from Charles River (Calco, Como, Italy) were used. The animals were housed according to Directive 2010/63/EU of the European Parliament and the Council and the WMA Statement on Animal Use in Biomedical Research. All procedures followed the guidelines of the animal care and use committee of the University of Bologna (Bologna, Italy) ("Protocol 2DBFE.N.YEV" by the Comitato Etico Scientifico for Animal Research Protocols according to D.L. vo 116/92 and approved by the Ministry of Health in December 2023). The animals were sacrificed by cervical dislocation, and the organs required were set up rapidly under a suitable resting tension in a 15 mL organ bath containing appropriate physiological salt solution (PSS) warmed and buffered to pH 7.4 by saturation with 95% O_2–5% CO_2 gas and used as described below.

Guinea pig gastric fundus. As previously described [46], the stomach was removed, opened along the mesentery of the greater curvature, and rinsed with Krebs bicarbonate-buffered solution maintained at 37 °C. Fundus muscle strips were cut parallel to the circular muscle layer, tied at each end with sutures, and hung in the organ baths containing Krebs bicarbonate-buffered solution.

Guinea pig ileum. The terminal portion of the ileum (3–4 cm near the ileo–caecal junction) was cleaned, and segments 2–3 cm long of ileum were set up under 1 g tension at 37 °C in organ baths containing Tyrode solution of the following composition (mM): NaCl, 118; KCl, 4.75; $CaCl_2$, 2.54; $mgSO_4 \cdot 7H_2O$, 1.20; $KH_2PO_4 \cdot 2H_2O$, 1.19; $NaHCO_3$ 25; and glucose 11. The two segments obtained (2–3 cm) were set up under 1 g tension in the longitudinal direction along the intestinal wall. Tissues were allowed to equilibrate for at least 30 min, during which the bathing solution was changed every 10 min.

Guinea pig proximal colon. Starting approximately 1 cm distal from the caecocolonic junction, two segments of about 1 cm of the guinea pig's proximal colon were cut. The proximal colon was cleaned by rinsing with De Jalon solution of the following composition (mM): NaCl, 155; KCl, 5.6; $CaCl_2$, 0.5; $NaHCO_3$, 6.0; and glucose, 2.8; and the mesenteric tissue was removed. The two segments were suspended in organ baths containing gassed, warm De Jalon solution under a load of 1 g maintained at 37 °C. Tension changes in longitudinal muscle length were recorded. Tissues were allowed to equilibrate for at least 30 min, during which the bathing solution was changed every 10 min.

Guinea pig heart. After thoracotomy, the heart was immediately removed and washed by perfusion through the aorta with oxygenated Tyrode solution of the following composition (mM): 136.9 NaCl, 5.4 KCl, 2.5 $CaCl_2$, 1.0 $mgCl_2$, 0.4 $NaH_2PO_4xH_2O$, 11.9 $NaHCO_3$, and 5.5 glucose. The physiological salt solution (PSS) was buffered at pH 7.4 by saturation with 95% O_2–5% CO_2 gas, and the temperature was maintained at 35 °C. The following isolated guinea pig heart preparations were used: spontaneously beating right atria and left atria driven at 1 Hz. For each preparation, the left and right atria were dissected from the ventricles, cleaned of excess tissue, and hung vertically in a 15 mL organ bath containing the described PSS. The contractile activity was recorded isometrically using a force transducer (FT 0.3, Grass Instruments Corporation, Quincy, MA, USA) using Power Lab® 8/30 software (AD-Instruments Pty Ltd., Castle Hill, Australia). The left atria were stimulated by rectangular pulses of 0.6–0.8 ms duration and about 50% threshold voltage through two platinum contact electrodes in the lower holding clamp (Grass S88 Stimulator).

The right atria were in spontaneous activity. After the tissues were beaten for several minutes, a length-tension curve was determined, and the muscle length was maintained at that, which elicited 90% of the maximum contractile force observed at the optimal length. A 45–60 min stabilization period was allowed before various agents challenged the atria. During the equilibration period, the bathing solution was changed every 15 min. The method to test inotropy and chronotropic activities was previously described [47].

Guinea pig aortic strips. The aortic strips were prepared as previously described [48].

2.2.2. Spontaneous Contractility on the Ileum and Colon

As previously described [44], the tracing graphs of spontaneous contractions of the gastric fundus, ileum, and proximal colon were continuously recorded with the LabChart 7.0 Pro Software (ADInstruments, Bella Vista, NSW, Australia). After the equilibration period (about 30 to 45 min according to each tissue), cumulative concentration curves (0.1, 0.5, 1, 5, and 10 mg/mL) to HEMEO were constructed. At the end of each single dose, the following parameters were evaluated considering a 5 min stationary period:

- Mean contraction amplitude (MCA), evaluated as the mean force value (g);
- Standard deviations of the force values over the period as an index of the spontaneous contraction variability (SCV);
- Basal spontaneous motor activity (BSMA), as the percentage (%) variation in each mean force value (g) for the control period;
- Spontaneous contractions were investigated in the frequency domain through a standard FFT analysis and a subsequent power spectral density (PSD) plot. The absolute powers of the following frequency bands of interest: low [0.0, 0.2] Hz (LF), medium [0.2, 0.6] Hz (MF), and high [0.6, 1.0] Hz (HF) [49], were then calculated.

The Lab Chart 7 Pro Software performed all the calculations in a post-processing phase. A skilled operator chose the analysis period to avoid errors due to artifacts.

2.2.3. Induced Contractility

Intestinal histamine receptor. As previously described, the H_1-receptor non-competitive antagonism activity of HEMEO was tested using guinea pig ileum [49]. Briefly, after a stabilization period, concentration–response curves were constructed by cumulative addition of the agonist (histamine). The agonist (histamine) concentration in the organ bath was added only after the response to the previous addition had attained a maximal level and remained steady. Contractions were recorded using a displacement transducer (FT. 03, Grass Instruments, Quincy, MA, USA) using Power Lab 7 Pro software (ADInstruments Pty Ltd., Castle Hill, Australia). In all cases, parallel experiments in which tissues received no antagonist were run to check any sensitivity variation. Concentration–response curves to agonist were obtained at 30 min intervals; the first was discarded, and the second was taken as control. Following incubation with the antagonist (HEMEO), a new concentration–response curve was obtained for the agonist. Tension changes were recorded isotonically.

2.2.4. Cardiovascular Guinea Pig Preparations

Heart histamine receptor. The H_2-receptor antagonism activity of HEMEO was tested using spontaneously beating right atria [50]. As previously described, after a stabilization period (see below), a cumulative dose–response curve to histamine (0.1–50 μM) was constructed. After washing out for 30 min, an incubation period (30 min) was conducted on the antagonist (HEMEO 0.5, 1, 5 mg/mL). Following incubation, a new curve for the agonist was constructed.

Inotropic and chronotropic activities. To test inotropic and chronotropic activities, the left atria were driven at 1 Hz and spontaneously beat the right atria following the previously described method [48]. After a stabilization period, experiments were carried out in both cases using a single concentration of HEMEO (1 mg/mL). Following incubation (30 min), a new curve for the agonist was constructed.

Spasmolytic activity on K^+ depolarized aortic strips. The thoracic aorta was excised and immersed in Tyrode solution with the following composition (in mM): 118 NaCl, 4.75 KCl, 2.54 $CaCl_2$, 1.20 $mgSO_4$, 1.19 KH_2PO_4, 25 $NaHCO_3$, and 11 glucose. The solution was equilibrated with a gas mixture of 95% O_2 and 5% CO_2, maintaining a pH of 7.4. After the equilibration period, guinea pig aortic strips were contracted by exposure to a physiological saline solution (PSS) containing 80 mM KCl, achieved through equimolar substitution of K^+ for Na^+. Tension changes in smooth muscle K^+ 80 mM-induced contraction were recorded isometrically as previously reported [48]. The effect of HEMEO was checked by constructing a cumulative concentration–effect curve.

2.2.5. Statistical Analysis

Experiments were performed in duplicate with tissue from the same animal, and mean values were recorded. The data presented are means ± SEM for a series of experiments with four animals for the gastric fundus and ileum and four to six animals for the proximal colon. Normality was assessed with the Shapiro–Wilk test.

Spontaneous contractility: Comparisons between mean spontaneous contraction amplitudes (MCAs) at different concentrations were performed by one-way ANOVA with Bonferroni's correction after assessing the data normality through a Kolgomorov–Smirnov test. Differences with $p < 0.05$ were considered statistically significant.

Since statistical analysis results on spontaneous motility are certainly accurate but too sensitive compared to the natural physiological behavior of the tissues, we hypothesized a personal classification scale that considers the percentage changes in the measured parameters compared to baseline values. Thus, the PSD% variations for each band of interest to control were estimated. LF, MF, and HF contractions were considered physiologically relevant when higher or lower than 50% variations for the basal values.

LF, MF, and HF percentage variations were classified depending on their value following these criteria: ≤−500%: "---"; [−500%, −300%]: "--"; [−300%,−50%]: "-"; [−50%, +50%]: "="; [+50%, +300%]: "+"; [+300%, +500%]: "++"; ≥+500%: "+++".

Similarly, tone variations were categorized as follows: ≤−100%: "------"; [−100%, −80%]: "-----"; [−80%, −60%]: "----"; [−60%, −40%]: "---"; [−40%, −20%]: "--"; [−20%, 0%]: "-"; Not significant: "="; [0%, +20%]: "+"; [+20%, +40%]: "++"; [+40%, +60%]: "+++"; [60%, +80%]: "++++"; [+80%, +100%]: "+++++"; ≥+100%: "++++++".

Induced contractility: the spasmolytic activity of samples was expressed as the percent inhibition of calcium-induced contraction on K^+-depolarized gastric fundus, ileum, colon, and aorta strips (smooth muscle activity). Data were analyzed by Student's t-test. The potency of all samples defined as IC_{50} was evaluated from log concentration–response curves (Probit analysis by Litchfield and Wilcoxon, n = 6–8) in the appropriate pharmacological preparations. All data are presented as mean ± SEM [51–53].

Determination of Dissociation Constants. In functional experiments, the antagonism activity to histamine of HEMEO was estimated by determining the concentration of the non-competitive antagonist that inhibited 50% of the maximum response to the agonist. Three different antagonist concentrations were used, each tested at least four times. A pharmacological computer program [51] was used to analyze the data. A p value less than 0.05 was considered significant. All the figures were created using GraphPad software v6.0 [52].

2.3. *Antimicrobial Disc Diffusion Test*

The agar disk diffusion method assessed the antimicrobial activity of the tested compounds against *Helicobacter pylori*. All solutions/suspensions were tested in parallel, using *H. pylori* G27 strain. Bacterial cells were recovered from glycerol stocks on Brucella broth agar plates containing 5% fetal calf serum (FCS), added with Dent's antibiotic supplement. Plates were incubated in a CO_2-controlled (9% CO_2) incubator (Thermo Scientific, Waltham, MA, USA) at 37 °C.

H. pylori cells were then collected from plates and resuspended in 0.5 mL of liquid Brucella broth with 5% FCS, and the cell density (OD_{600}) of bacterial suspension was determined. Then, bacteria were diluted in melted Brucella broth Soft Agar medium (Brucella broth agar plates containing 0.5% agar) to obtain a final OD_{600} of 0.07, and 6.5 mL of this suspension was poured onto a sterile standard Brucella broth agar plate. After that, sterile paper discs (diameter of 5 mm) were deposited onto the agar plates.

For HEMEO, two concentrations were prepared in sterile water and tested (100 mg/mL and 20 mg/mL). Then, 4 µL of the tested compounds was dropped on the disc. The H_2O vehicle solutions were used as the negative control, while Kanamycin (2.5 mg/mL in H_2O) was used as the reference antibiotic. The plates were incubated under microaerophilic conditions at 37 °C for 72 h; then, the diameter of the inhibition zone was measured. This experiment was performed in biological triplicates, and the average inhibition diameter was calculated for each tested concentration [54].

2.4. Antioxidant Capacity Assay

The FRAP assay evaluated the antioxidant capacity of HEMEO according to Benzie et al. [55]. Briefly, different amounts of compounds were added to the FRAP reagent solution, and the formation of the Fe^{2+}–tripyridyltriazine complex was monitored spectrophotometrically at λ 595 nm, T = 30 °C, at time 0 (Abs0), and after 3 min (Abs3) using a Jasco V-750 spectrophotometer equipped with a stirring device and thermostatic control. Standard Fe^{2+} was used for the calibration curve. Data are expressed as ΔAbs (Abs3 − Abs0) on mg. All measurements were performed in triplicate ± SD.

3. Results

3.1. HEMEO Essential Oils Components Qualitative Profile

To verify the persistence of the three selected essential oils in HEMEO, a GC-MS qualitative analysis of the dichloromethane extracts obtained from the formulated mixture was undertaken. The investigation focused on detecting the most characteristic terpenes of the three essential oils, i.e., trans-anethole, menthol, and estragole (Figures S1–S3, Supplementary Materials). The selected terpenes were unambiguously identified by comparison with the retention time of standard solutions and by their MS spectra using the library (NIST version 2.4) for comparison. In particular, trans-anethole (Figure S1) confirmed the presence of *Pimpinella anisum* and *Foeniculum vulgare* [56,57] as it is the principal and most characteristic terpene in these essential oils; in addition, estragole (Figure S2), a phenylpropanoid typically contained in fennel, was a further hint of the persistence of *Pimpinella anisum* in the formulation [57,58]. Eventually, menthol (Figure S3) was detected, and the presence of *Mentha piperita* essential oil [59] was ascertained. The peak area of the characteristic terpenes was reasonably assumed to be the response to assess the stability of the essential oils. The peak area RSD% (n = 9) measured at the time of product preparation and after 3, 6, and 12 months of storage under conventional conditions (closed, room temperature, dark) was <5.2% (n = 9).

As expected, several minor components were observed in the chromatograms due to the presence of the other terpenes of the essential oils and the volatile components of the formulation; interestingly, the selected terpenes were the most represented, demonstrating that the adopted formulation allows for embedding the essential oils, ensuring their stability during storage.

3.2. Total Phenolic Content (TPC) of HEMEO

The TPC of HEMEO was quantified using the Folin–Ciocalteu assay. As shown in Table 1, the result expressed as mg of gallic acid equivalent (GAE) per g of HEMEO was 9.925 ± 0.42 mg GAE/g HEMEO (n = 5).

Table 1. HEMEO total phenolic content (TPC).

Concentration	TPC [a]
HEMEO	9.925 ± 0.42

[a] Total phenolic content, expressed as mg gallic acid equivalent GAE/g (n = 5) HEMEO.

3.3. Ex Vivo Studies

Spontaneous contractility. The effect of HEMEO on the spontaneous contractility of the gastric fundus, ileum, and colon were studied. Figures 3–5 show the effects of HEMEO on the longitudinal stomach, ileum, and colon muscles' spontaneous contractility.

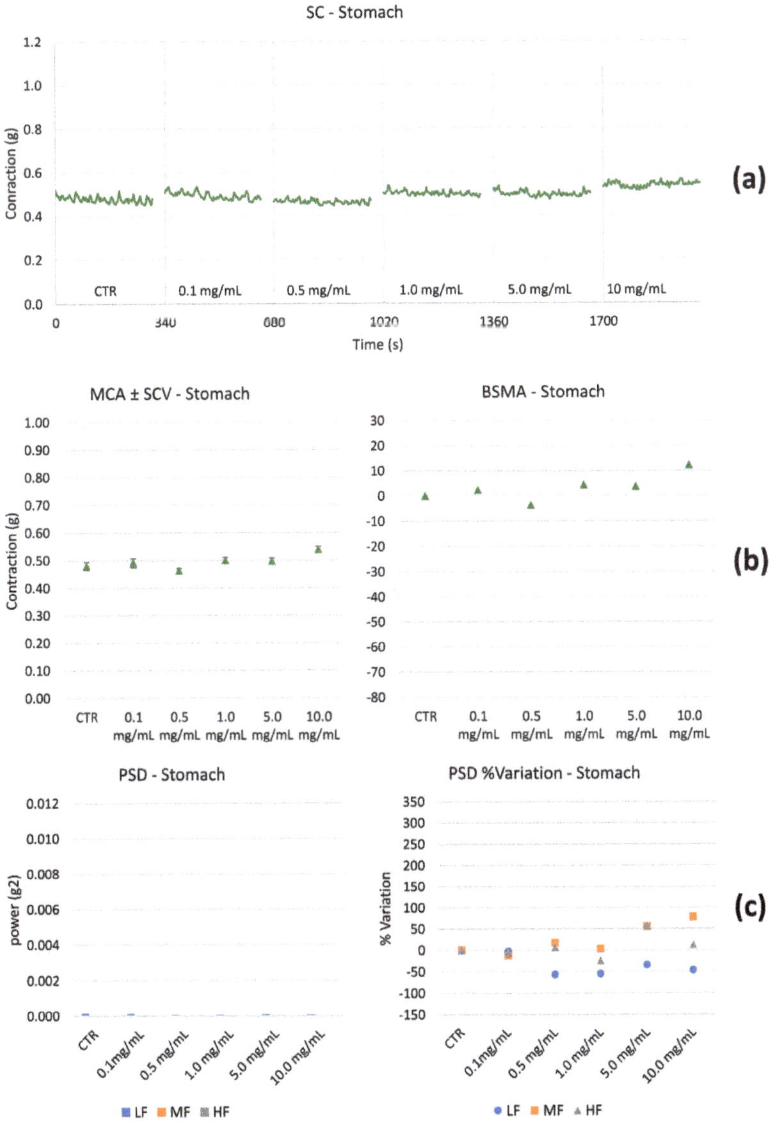

Figure 3. Example of experimental original recording of the concentration–response curve of HEMEO on spontaneous longitudinal (Long) stomach basal contractility. (**a**) Spontaneous contraction (SC) signals

for each concentration; (**b**) mean contraction amplitude (MCA) and spontaneous contraction variability (SCV), represented as error bars in the MCA plot and contraction percentage variation for the control (BSMA) for each considered condition; all the comparisons resulted in being statistically significant ($p < 0.05$); (**c**) power spectral density (PSD) and percentage variations. Despite statistically significant differences between muscular tones at different HEMEO concentrations, the MCA variations are not physiologically significant (less than 20%). MF and HF bands values increase over 50% only for concentrations of 5.0 mg/mL and 10 mg/mL, suggesting a slight increase in mixing and pain.

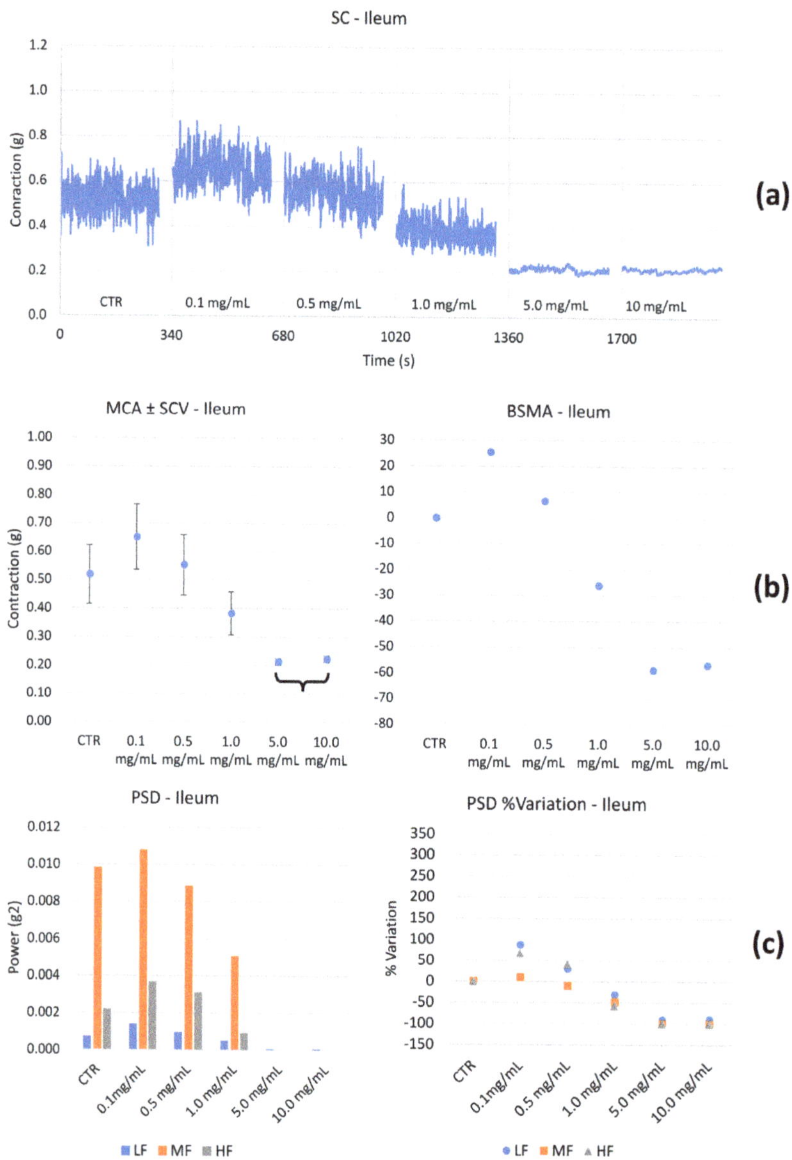

Figure 4. Example of experimental original recording of the concentration–response curve of HEMEO on spontaneous longitudinal (Long) ileum basal contractility. (**a**) Spontaneous contraction (SC) signals

for each concentration; (**b**) mean contraction amplitude (MCA) and spontaneous contraction variability (SCV), represented as error bars in the MCA plot and contraction percentage variation for the control (BSMA) for each considered condition; not statistically significant differences ($p > 0.05$) between MCAs at different concentrations are reported in the graph with a curly bracket. All the comparisons not reported are to be considered significant ($p < 0.05$); (**c**) power spectral density (PSD) and percentage variations. Longitudinal tones present a biphasic behavior: it increases for 0.1 mg/mL concentrations and then decreases until a maximum difference of −60%. LF and HF present the same tend.

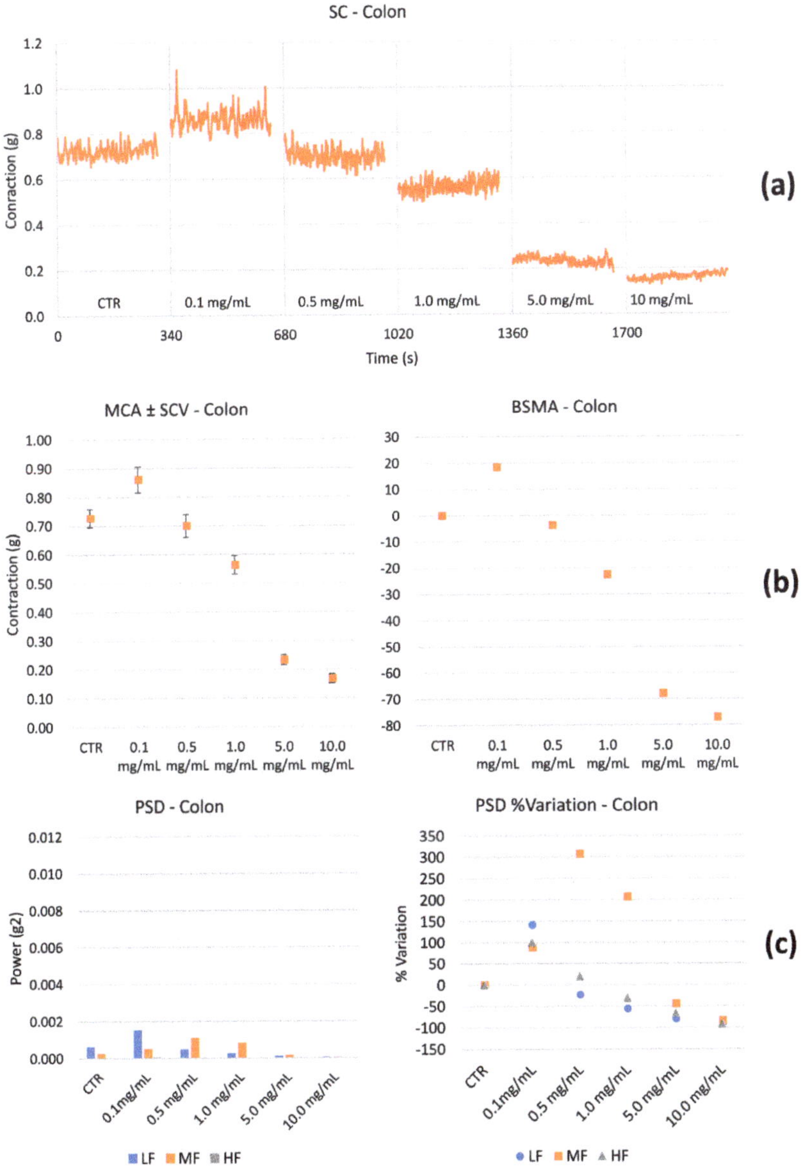

Figure 5. Example of experimental original recording of the concentration–response curve of HEMEO on spontaneous longitudinal (Long) colon basal contractility. (**a**) Spontaneous contraction (SC) signals

for each concentration; (**b**) mean contraction amplitude (MCA) and spontaneous contraction variability (SCV), represented as error bars in the MCA plot and contraction percentage variation for the control (BSMA) for each considered condition; all the comparisons reported resulted statistically significant ($p < 0.05$); (**c**) power spectral density (PSD) and percentage variations. Longitudinal tones present a biphasic behavior: it increases for 0.1 mg/mL concentrations and then decreases until a maximum difference of −80%. LF and HF bands present the same biphasic trend. MF has a maximum increase of 300% at 0.5 mg/mL, then decreases after 5.0 mg/mL.

Stomach: HEMEO effect on the longitudinal contractions of the stomach does not show physiologically significant effects on BSCA. The PSD percentage (%) variations for LF are not significant; differences in MF and HF contractions are significant only for the higher concentrations.

Based on our previous experience [60], LF related to the longitudinal smooth muscle is linked to transit speed: the higher the PSD band, the higher the transit speed. MF and HF are likely associated with pain. This last hypothesis was already proposed in the present study and verified for the ileum and colon; the same mechanism must be demonstrated for the stomach. Table 2 summarizes the results obtained; LF, MF, and HF were not significantly different in the stomach. Therefore, it can be argued that HEMEO does not modify tone and transit time, and its antibacterial activity could be carried out without the limit of accelerated emptying. The ileum and colon showed similar behavior. At low concentrations, transit velocity, pain, and tone increased. The parameters decreased for concentrations greater than or equal to 1.0 mg/mL (Tables S1–S6).

Table 2. Effects on stomach, ileum, and colon of HEMEO, including transit speed, pain, and muscle tones.

	Stomach					Ileum					Colon				
mg/mL	0.1	0.5	1.0	5.0	10.0	0.1	0.5	1.0	5.0	10.0	0.1	0.5	1.0	5.0	10.0
Transit speed variation%	=	-	-	=	=	+	=	=	-	-	+	=	-	-	-
Pain%	=	=	=	+	+	+	=	-	-	-	+	=	=	-	-
Longitudinal contraction variation%	=	=	=	=	=	++	+	--	---	---	+	-	--	----	----

Percentage variations in transit speed and pain: "—": ≤−500%; "–": [−500%, −300%]; "-": [−300%, −50%]; "=": [−50%, +50%]; "+": [+50%, +300%]; "++": [+300%, +500%]; Percentage contraction variations: "—-": [−80%, −60%]; "—": [−60%, −40%]; "–": [−40%, −20%]; "-": [−20%, 0%]; "=": Not significant; "+": [0%, +20%]; "++": [+20%, +40%].

Histamine receptors. HEMEO was evaluated for its ability to modulate the activity of gut H_1-histamine receptors. The H_1 subtype in the gastrointestinal system contributes to the control of contractility [60], while the H_2 subtype is prevalent in cardiac tissue, where it modulates heart rate [61]. Table 3 and Figure 6 show that HEMEO antagonizes histamine-induced contraction on the ileum in a non-competitive mechanism. These effects were reversible with 30 min of washing. The same study, conducted on the H_2-histaminic receptor of cardiac tissue, gave a negative result: HEMEO (1 mg/mL) did not modify the increase in heart rate induced by histamine.

Table 3. Histamine receptor activity of HEMEO.

Ileum [a]		Right Atrium [b]	
IC_{50} [c]	95% Conf-Lim.	IC_{50} [c]	95% Conf-Lim.
0.78	0.66–0.87	#	

[a] Guinea pig ileum smooth muscle. [b] Guinea pig spontaneously beating right atrium [c] The inhibition concentration (IC_{50}) was expressed as mg/mL concentration and was calculated from concentration–response curves (Probit analysis by Litchfield and Wilcoxon with n = 5–6) [51]. # inactive up to 5 mg/mL.

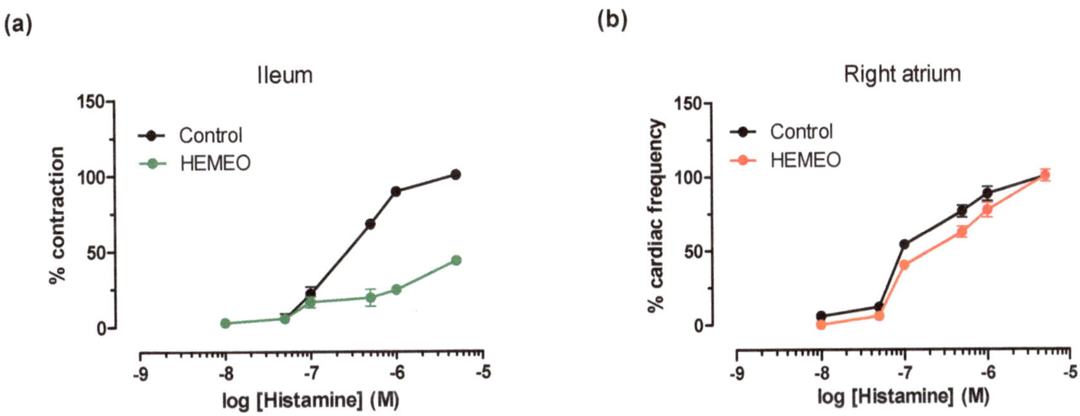

Figure 6. Effect of HEMEO on histamine-induced contraction in isolated guinea pig ileum (**a**) and in spontaneously beating right atrium (**b**). Cumulative concentration–response curves were obtained before and after exposure to HEMEO (1 mg/mL) for 30 min. Each point is the mean ± SEM (n = 5–6). Where error bars are not shown, these are covered by the point itself.

Calcium Channels. HEMEO effect on selected gastrointestinal tracts (gastric fundus, ileum, and colon) was evaluated to verify its potential spasmolytic effects on K^+-induced contraction; the considered tracts had fundamental involvement in the digestive process. In addition, the effects of HEMEO were evaluated on guinea pig aorta smooth muscle. The obtained data are shown in Table 4. As can be seen, HEMEO did not inhibit potassium-induced stomach contraction; it showed a concentration-dependent spasmolytic action on the ileum and colon, with approximately four times greater potency on the ileum concerning the colon. In addition, the maximum concentration (10 mg/mL) on the aorta suggested a weak contractile effect.

Table 4. Spasmolytic effect of HEMEO on smooth muscle preparations.

Tissue	IA [a]	IC_{50} [b]	95% Conf-Lim.
Gastric Fundus	24.0 ± 2.6		
Ileum	63.0 ± 3.7	1.33	1.11–1.60
Colon	98.0 ± 1.3	5.31	4.84–5.84
Aorta	12.0 ± 0.3 [c]		

[a] Intrinsic activity (IA) expressed as percent inhibition of calcium-induced contraction on K^+-depolarized (80 mM) guinea pig gastric fundus, ileum, colon, and aortic strips at 10 mg/mL. Data are presented as M ± S.E.M. [b] The 50% of the effect of concentration (IC_{50}) was expressed as mg/mL and calculated from concentration–response curves (Probit analysis by Litchfield and Wilcoxon [51] with n = 6–7). When the maximum effect was <50%, the IC_{50} values were not calculated. [c] positive effect.

Cardiac parameters. The cardiac profile of HEMEO was assessed at 1 mg/mL concentration on guinea pig isolated left and right atria, driven at 1 Hz to evaluate the inotropic effect. The chronotropic activity was also assessed by spontaneously beating the right atrium. The obtained data related to 1 h of incubation are shown in Table 5. HEMEO did not modify the force of cardiac contraction evaluated on the left atrium driven at 1 Hz and on the spontaneously beating right atrium, and it had no effects on the heart rate monitored on the right atrium in spontaneous activity.

Table 5. Cardiac activity of HEMEO.

Left Atrium	Right Atrium	
Negative Inotropy [a]	Negative Inotropy [b]	Negative Chronotropy
IA [a]	IA [b]	IA [c]
*	*	*

[a,b] IA: intrinsic activity expressed as a decrease in developed tension on isolated guinea pig left atrium driven at 1 Hz and on guinea pig spontaneously beating right atrium at 1 mg/mL HEMEO concentration, expressed as percent change from the control (*n* = 5–6). [c] Decrease in the atrial rate of HEMEO (1 mg/mL) on guinea pig spontaneously beating right atrium. Pretreatment heart rate ranged from 165 to 190 beats/min. * inactive.

3.4. Antioxidant Activity

The antioxidant capacity of HEMEO was evaluated using the FRAP assay, revealing a dose–response relationship with the different concentrations of HEMEO tested (Figure 7a). Specifically, a 1 mg/mL concentration of HEMEO generated a FRAP signal comparable to that produced by 8.3 µg/mL (equivalent to 47 nM) of ascorbate, used as a reference antioxidant compound (Figure 7b). The IC_{50} of HEMEO was estimated to be about 0.25 mg/mL).

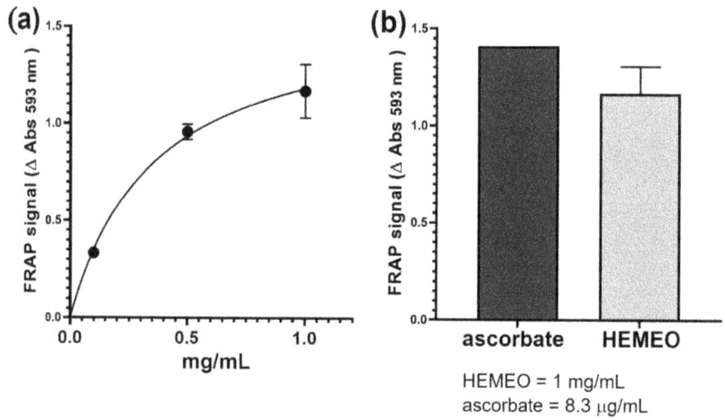

Figure 7. (**a**) The antioxidant power of the HEMEO solution was measured using the FRAP assay. (**b**) Comparison of 1 mg/mL HEMEO antioxidant power with the reference compound ascorbate.

3.5. Antimicrobial Activity

To assess the antimicrobial activity of HEMEO against *H. pylori*, a disk diffusion assay was performed using HEMEO (80 µg/disk) on Brucella Broth agar, incubated at 37 °C for 72 h. The mean zone of inhibition was 12 ± 2 mm, while negative control disks (solvent only) produced no inhibition, confirming compound activity (Table 6, Figure S4). The activity profile was similar to the reference antibiotic Kanamycin, even if the potency was considerably lower (Kanamycin, at a concentration of 2.5 mg/mL, inhibits growth by 35 ± 2). The results obtained in our assay align well with those reported for other extracts and preparations of similar complexity tested against *H. pylori* using the same methodology [62–66].

Table 6. HEMEO and positive control vs. *H. pylori* G27.

Sample	Concentration			
	2.5 mg/mL [a]	20.0 mg/mL [a]	100 mg/mL [a]	MAQ [b]
HEMEO	NT	12 ± 2	22 ± 4	20.0
Karnamicyn	35 ± 2	NT	NT	

[a] Mean diameter of inhibition (mm ± SD). [b] MAQ (minimum active quantity) values expressed as mg/mL of samples tested for activity against *H. pylori* G27.

4. Discussion

HEMEO is an herbal mixture containing three essential oils formulated to harness the synergistic effects of various organic compounds that can simultaneously target multiple pathways associated with specific pathologies [15]. The native liquid state of the essential oils is suitable for most applications. However, the solid form is preferred when intended to be used as a component in oral dosage nutraceutical formulations. In HEMEO, conventional excipients such as silica were used to deliver the essential oils of *Foeniculum vulgare* Mill, *Mentha piperita* L., and *Pimpinella anisum* L. The results of the GC-MS analysis carried out on the formulation at different storage times demonstrated the stability of the HEMEO solid formulation.

By combining multiple herbs, HEMEO extends its therapeutic effects to a broader spectrum of conditions than it would with a single herb. Lowering the individual herb concentrations required may also help reduce off-target effects, decreasing the likelihood of unintended interactions with proteins or other molecular targets beyond the intended scope [58].

The chemical profile of HEMEO guided this study's focus on its potential application in managing gastrointestinal contractility disorders, an essential aspect of many gastrointestinal conditions [67].

Peristaltic waves typically propel chyme along short segments of the intestine rather than the entire tract. However, the regulation of intestinal propulsion relies on the brain–gut axis, which is influenced by both extrinsic innervation (splanchnic and vagal–sacral pathways) and intrinsic networks (the myenteric and *submucosal plexi*). Much of the knowledge about gastrointestinal contractility comes from studies focused on specific GI regions or animal models, and these indicate that motility regulation mechanisms vary by anatomical site and muscle type. The expression of receptors, mechanisms for smooth muscle excitability, and regulation of contractile force all contribute to a highly complex brain–gut interaction system. A further challenge is that motility disorders may be localized, manifesting in specific gastrointestinal tract segments but not others. For example, hypomotility in the colon may lead to constipation without significantly affecting other segments. As a result, treatments aimed at increasing motility in one area risk inadvertently disrupting motility elsewhere [68]. A schematic diagram showing the detailed mechanism by which polyherbal extract protects against intestinal motility disorders is illustrated in Figure 8.

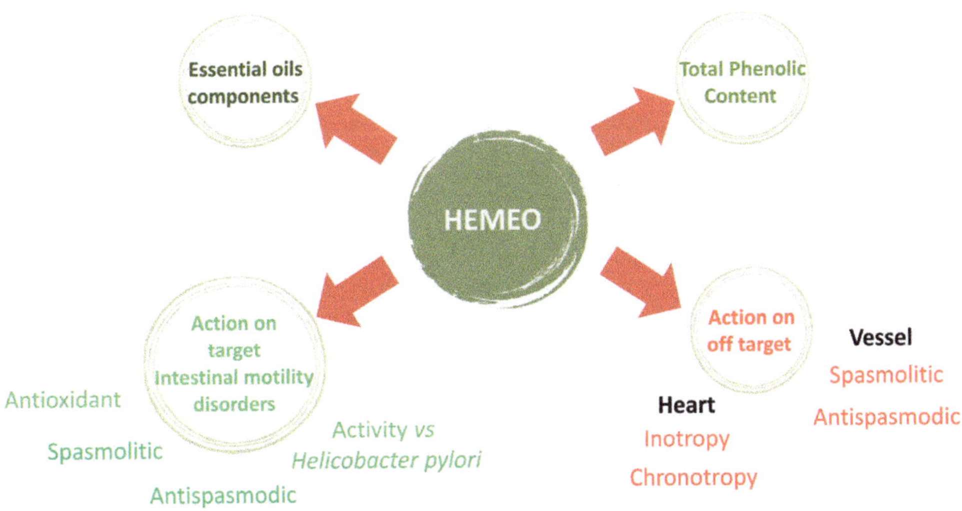

Figure 8. Schematic diagram showing the detail of the experimental design.

To evaluate the HEMEO activity, three key digestive processes—the stomach, ileum, and colon—were examined, assessing the effects on spontaneous and induced contractility and the outer layers of the guinea pig gut muscular tissues. The guinea pig is a well-known model for human intestinal studies and microbiome research and is predictive of translation to humans [69].

The latter contributes to contracting, relaxing, shortening, and lengthening the gut, providing the forces necessary to stir the gut contents and move food, water, and waste through the tubular chambers in one direction. The contractility of the longitudinal muscle is illustrated in the baseline of Figures 3–5. The propulsion of the ingesta farther down the gastrointestinal tract is contributed by the segmenting contractions of the outer longitudinal muscle. HEMEO has been shown to not significantly affect the spontaneous contractility of the stomach at the low doses studied.

It is known that decreasing gastric smooth muscle tone may decrease symptoms induced by gastric filling in patients with gastric accommodation, improving functional dyspeptic symptoms due to the reduction in gastric tone and increased compliance following ingestion of a meal. Transit speed, pain, and tone were increased in the ileum at low doses (HEMEO at 0.1–0.5 mg/mL), but no effect was observed at high doses. In the colon, tone, transit speed, and pain increased at the lowest dose but remained unchanged or decreased at higher doses. The decrease in transit velocity suggests a longer residence time of the intestinal contents and, therefore, better mixing/absorption/digestion/enzymatic work in the ileum. The two maximal doses of HEMEO were significantly different from the base, and a biphasic trend was observed: at low doses, MCA and SCV increased, whereas, at the higher doses, the observed values were lower than the control. The decrease in tone is associated with a relaxation of the smooth muscle fibers, leading to a global improvement in the digestive process and less pain in the colon. For example, IBS, a well-known intestinal disorder, is associated with diverse pathophysiological mechanisms, including increased abnormal colonic motility or transit. HEMEO, at the high doses applied in the present study, was found to decrease pain, tone, and transit, suggesting that it could serve as a supportive treatment for increased abnormal colonic motility or transit and relieve pain in IBS (Table 2).

The biphasic effect observed with HEMEO may be attributed to the involvement of different receptor populations, as described in the literature for conventional drugs [70]. In the case of HEMEO, a blend of herbal extracts and essential oils, effects on multiple targets are highly plausible.

Regarding its effect on calcium movements in the gastrointestinal tract, HEMEO has shown a spasmolytic effect on potassium-induced contractions [71]. While 1,4-Dihydropyridines primarily target vascular muscles, thus limiting their use in intestinal motility control [72], otilonium bromide selectively affects intestinal smooth muscles [73]. Therefore, it proves helpful in inflammatory intestinal diseases and cannot affect heart parameters [49,74,75]. HEMEO selectively affects the ileum and colon without interfering with stomach contractility, and its lack of effect on vascular smooth muscle positions it as an off-target therapeutic option.

These results support HEMEO's potential use in managing stomach atony. At the appropriate dose, HEMEO (Table 6) can control the growth of *H. pylori* while supporting healthy digestive function. *H. pylori* contributes to digestive disruptions. Once thought to be almost sterile due to its high acidity, the stomach hosts microorganisms, primarily *Firmicutes* [76]. In addition, proteolytic enzymes transform macronutrients into more easily absorbable molecules, proving to be an effective barrier against infections [77].

However, the environment allows for the growth of *H. pylori* microorganisms that can live and replicate at low pH values. In turn, *H. pylori* implements a series of mechanisms to modify the pH, making the surrounding environment alkaline and creating favorable conditions for its survival. *H. pylori* is primarily implicated in gastric diseases but has also been associated with various systemic conditions [11]. *H. pylori* infection triggers a series of events, including inflammation and reduction in secretory capacity, which leads to a clinical picture called atrophic gastritis [78]. *H. pylori* is also implicated in the onset of peptic ulcers by producing particular toxins that cause damage to the gastric epithelium associated with gastric diseases and cancer [79].

Clinical investigations have shown that *H. pylori* infection and the concomitant use of NSAIDs or acetylsalicylic acid increase the risk of peptic ulcer compared to patients who were proven to be susceptible to the infection [80].

All these insults produced by *H pylori* on the gastric wall highlight its essential role in the cascade leading to cancer development [81]. Conventional therapy involves using a combination of antibiotics and proton pump inhibitors [82]. The resistance to antibiotics induced by the continual use of conventional therapy has driven interest in the search for natural alternatives that can contribute to the control of this microorganism, suggesting the use of foods or plant extracts with proven action against *H pylori,* acting mainly through the inhibition of specific enzymatic pathways [83]. Among these, green tea chains and polyphenols such as the gingerols of *Zingiber officinalis* and essential oils such as those obtained from peppermint [84] have aroused interest.

HEMEO contains peppermint essential oils whose volatile compounds are known for their antibacterial action against this microorganism, contributing to the action of HEMEO on the *H. pylori* target [85]. The essential oil of *Pimpinella anisum,* rich in anethole, inhibits the growth of *H. Pylori* while simultaneously inhibiting the expression of COX-2 [86]. The literature describes the positive effects of combining *Glycyrrhiza glabra* with antibiotics [87]. At a concentration of 20 mg/mL, HEMEO inhibits the growth of *H pylori,* contributing to the maintenance of gastric function and exercising a protective role. In this case, the presence of *Glycyrrhiza glabra* increases the effectiveness of the mix. Still, the simultaneous presence of other extracts allows for the reduction in the concentration of *Glycyrrhiza glabra* phytocoplex, avoiding the known effects on the cardiovascular system, which represents an off-target effect [88]. Moreover, glycyrrhizin, a component of *Glycyrrhiza glabra,* has been shown to promote gastric mucosal healing, while glycyrrhizic acid exhibits spasmolytic effects, helping to alleviate gastrointestinal discomfort [89,90]. In our study, HEMEO exhibited a mild contractile impact, reaching a maximum of 12% at a concentration of 10 mg/mL, selectively acting on smooth muscles of the ileum and colon without compromising cardiac function. This selective action may provide a therapeutic advantage by targeting gastrointestinal motility without triggering systemic cardiovascular effects, which is significant given the cardiovascular side effects often associated with *Glycyrrhiza glabra* at higher concentrations. Moreover, other plant species, such as *Tabebuia,* have demonstrated anti-*H. pylori* properties [81].

Scientific literature has demonstrated that patients with *H. pylori* infection who are treated with L-type calcium channel blockers have a lower risk of developing gastric cancer [91]. HEMEO interferes with calcium movements similarly to well-known calcium modulators in cardiovascular [72] and gastrointestinal disorders [49,92].

In addition to its role in calcium modulation, HEMEO provides gastrointestinal support by incorporating *Asparagus racemosus* and *Foeniculum vulgare* essential oils, each contributing specific properties relevant to gastrointestinal health. *Asparagus racemosus* Willd. Oberm, an herbaceous plant from the *Lamiaceae* family, is predominantly used as a urinary antiseptic due to its methyl mercaptan content [93]. In Ayurvedic medicine, the roots are considered stomachic, and the extract is utilized in preparations for peptic ulcers [22], including those induced by prolonged ranitidine use [24], owing to its antimicrobial [23] and antifungal properties [94]. Studies by Bhatnagar et al. demonstrate that using *Asparagus racemosus* is associated with significant antidiarrheal activity by inhibiting intestinal motility [27]. Additionally, *Asparagus* is known for its detoxifying properties: Ayurvedic medicine traditionally uses this herb to purify the body and enhance overall health. It supports the elimination of toxins and promotes kidney function, thereby contributing to the body's natural detoxification processes [95,96].

Foeniculum vulgare Mill, commonly known as fennel, is used in traditional medicine to treat various conditions, particularly digestion and respiration [34]. Traditional practices emphasize its antimicrobial and antifungal activities, confirmed for both aqueous extracts of aerial parts [35] and essential oil [36]. The essential oil from the seeds also exhibits hepatoprotective properties, likely due to *d-limonene* and *β-myrcene* [37]. It contributes to regulating intestinal motility and relieving gastrointestinal atony or discomfort [97]. Additionally, anethole, an essential compound in fennel, has shown anticancer properties [98]. *Tabebuia avellanedae* is traditionally recognized for its detoxifying effects, particularly its ability to enhance the body's ability to eliminate toxins. Its compounds support liver function and promote overall health by purifying the blood and improving circulation. Recent studies highlight its antioxidant properties, contributing to immune system support and general well-being [99].

Histamine is present in the gastrointestinal system, especially during inflammatory processes. It is essential in numerous gastrointestinal pathologies, such as IBS. HEMEO modulates the histamine H_1 receptor in a reversible, non-competitive manner in the intestine without altering the heart rate (Table 3, Figure 6). This result is particularly interesting, as it allows for the modulation of intestinal contractility without off-target effects. Given that HEMEO is a blend of multiple extracts, the observed TPC likely reflects an additive or synergistic effect, resulting in a level slightly above that of individual plant extracts. This increased TPC may enhance the overall antioxidant potential of HEMEO compared to its components, suggesting a comprehensive approach to mitigating oxidative stress, which is a disrupted parameter in most diseases.

The TPC of HEMEO, measured at 9.925 mg GAE/g, and its antioxidant capacity, comparable to 8.3 μg/mL of ascorbic acid, place it within a favorable range for natural extracts and substantial for multi-component blends. This observation aligns with research on various Mediterranean plants, highlighting a solid relationship between TPC and antioxidant efficacy [100]. It indicates that even moderate levels of polyphenols can yield significant antioxidative effects.

A significant limitation of this study is the small sample size analyzed. Our primary focus was the methodological approach to accurately assess the biochemical, bacteriological, antioxidant, and motility-related aspects of gastric and intestinal tissues exposed to drug effects. Further investigations are required to delve deeper into the toxicological properties of herbal preparations [101,102] and the essential oils in HEMEO [103] to validate our findings and evaluate inter- and intra-individual variability.

5. Conclusions

The diverse range of activities demonstrated by HEMEO highlights its potential application in the formulation of dietary supplements targeting various health needs. Its selective effect on ileum and colon motility, as defined by the Rome Foundation criteria, suggests potential benefits in managing functional motility disorders associated with multiple pathologies [104]. Additionally, the mixed herbal extract, including essential oils, inhibits the growth of *Helicobacter pylori* without impairing spontaneous or induced stomach contractions.

The presence of specific bioactive compounds—such as saponins in *Asparagus racemosus*, flavonoids and glycyrrhizin in *Glycyrrhiza glabra*, menthol in *Mentha piperita*, and anethole in *Pimpinella anisum*—is central to HEMEO's therapeutic effects. These compounds, known for their anti-inflammatory, spasmolytic, antimicrobial, and antioxidant properties, significantly contribute to HEMEO's efficacy in disease prevention and as an adjunct in managing specific gastrointestinal conditions.

In summary, HEMEO represents a promising candidate for further research and development in dietary supplements. Its multifaceted properties offer notable therapeutic advantages [105].

Nevertheless, although extensive information exists on the effects of individual components, further in-depth studies are ongoing to evaluate HEMEO's effects in a translational context, particularly regarding its potential synergistic interactions with drugs [106].

Supplementary Materials: The supporting files can be downloaded at: https://www.mdpi.com/article/10.3390/nu16244357/s1, Figure S1: Total ion current GC chromatograms of a standard solution of trans-anethole (a) and dichloromethane extract from the real sample (b) and their on-line mass spectra: trans-anethole standard (c) and real sample (d). Chromatographic and detection conditions are reported in the text; Figure S2: Total ion current GC chromatograms of a standard solution of estragole (a) and dichloromethane extract from the real sample (b) and their on-line mass spectra: estragole standard (c) and real sample (d). Chromatographic and detection conditions are reported in the text; Figure S3: Total ion current GC chromatograms of a standard solution of menthol (a) and dichloromethane extract from the real sample (b) and their on-line mass spectra: menthol standard (c) and real sample (d). Chromatographic and detection conditions are reported in the text; Figure S4: Zone of inhibition; Table S1: Spontaneous motility data of stomach tissue; Table S2: Effect size (ANOVA with Bonferroni's correction) for stomach tissue; Table S3: Spontaneous motility data of ileum tissue; Table S4: Effect size (ANOVA with Bonferroni's correction) for ileum tissue; Table S5: Spontaneous motility data of colon tissue; Table S6: Effect size (ANOVA with Bonferroni's correction) for colon tissue.

Author Contributions: Conceptualization, R.B., L.B.M., I.C. and R.G.; methodology, M.M., S.R., C.B., N.R., D.R. and D.D.L.; investigation, L.B.M., N.R., I.C., R.S., D.D.L., S.R., C.M. and R.G.; validation, R.B., R.G. and L.B.M.; data curation, R.B., L.B.M., I.C., S.R. and C.M.; writing—original draft preparation, R.B., R.G. and L.B.M.; writing—review and editing, R.B., R.G., I.C. and L.B.M.; visualization, R.B., L.B.M. and R.G.; supervision, R.B., L.B.M. and R.G.; project administration, R.B., L.B.M. and R.G.; funding acquisition, R.B. All authors have read and agreed to the published version of the manuscript.

Funding: This work was supported by the 2022 (RFO) Ricerca Fondamentale Orientata–University of Bologna, Italy.

Institutional Review Board Statement: The animals were housed according to the ECC Council Directive regarding protecting animals for experimental and other scientific purposes (Directive 2010/63/EU of the European Parliament and of the Council) and the WMA Statement on Animal Use in Biomedical Research. All procedures followed the guidelines of the animal care and use committee of the University of Bologna (Bologna, Italy). The ethical committee authorization was reported and numbered as "Protocol 2DBFE.N.YEV" by the Comitato Etico Scientifico for Animal Research Protocols according to D.L. vo 116/92 and approved by the Ministry of Health in December 2023.

Informed Consent Statement: Not applicable.

Data Availability Statement: Data are available upon request to the corresponding author.

Conflicts of Interest: Authors Simone Roncioni, Roberta Scanferlato, Dalila De Luca and Carla Marzetti worked for Valsambro S.r.l. The remaining authors declare no conflicts of interest.

References

1. Cheng, L.K.; O'Grady, G.; Du, P.; Egbuji, J.U.; Windsor, J.A.; Pullan, A.J. Gastrointestinal System. *Wiley Interdiscip. Rev. Syst. Biol. Med.* **2010**, *2*, 65–79. [CrossRef] [PubMed]
2. Di Natale, M.R.; Athavale, O.N.; Wang, X.; Du, P.; Cheng, L.K.; Liu, Z.; Furness, J.B. Functional and Anatomical Gastric Regions and Their Relations to Motility Control. *Neurogastroenterol. Motil.* **2023**, *35*, e14560. [CrossRef] [PubMed]
3. Van Den Abeele, J.; Rubbens, J.; Brouwers, J.; Augustijns, P. The Dynamic Gastric Environment and Its Impact on Drug and Formulation Behaviour. *Eur. J. Pharm. Sci.* **2017**, *96*, 207–231. [CrossRef] [PubMed]
4. Abell, T.L.; Werkman, R.F. Gastrointestinal Motility Disorders. *Am. Fam. Physician* **1996**, *53*, 895–902. [PubMed]
5. Malagelada, J.R. The Brain-Gut Team. *Dig. Dis.* **2020**, *38*, 293–298. [CrossRef]
6. Tack, J.; Janssen, P. Gastroduodenal Motility. *Curr. Opin. Gastroenterol.* **2010**, *26*, 647–655. [CrossRef]
7. Camilleri, M. Management Options for Irritable Bowel Syndrome. *Mayo Clin. Proc.* **2018**, *93*, 1858–1872. [CrossRef]
8. Hunt, R.H.; Camilleri, M.; Crowe, S.E.; El-Omar, E.M.; Fox, J.G.; Kuipers, E.J.; Malfertheiner, P.; McColl, K.E.L.; Pritchard, D.M.; Rugge, M.; et al. The Stomach in Health and Disease. *Gut* **2015**, *64*, 1650–1668. [CrossRef]
9. Ghoshal, U.C. Marshall and Warren Lecture 2019: A Paradigm Shift in Pathophysiological Basis of Irritable Bowel Syndrome and Its Implication on Treatment. *J. Gastroenterol. Hepatol.* **2020**, *35*, 712–721. [CrossRef]
10. Burucoa, C.; Axon, A. Epidemiology of Helicobacter Pylori Infection. *Helicobacter* **2017**, *22* (Suppl. 1), e12403. [CrossRef]
11. Gravina, A.G.; Zagari, R.M.; De Musis, C.; Romano, L.; Loguercio, C.; Romano, M. Helicobacter Pylori and Extragastric Diseases: A Review. *World J. Gastroenterol.* **2018**, *24*, 3204–3221. [CrossRef] [PubMed]

12. Kountouras, J.; Polyzos, S.A.; Doulberis, M.; Zeglinas, C.; Artemaki, F.; Vardaka, E.; Deretzi, G.; Giartza-Taxidou, E.; Tzivras, D. Vlachaki, E.; et al. Potential Impact of Helicobacter Pylori-Related Metabolic Syndrome on Upper and Lower Gastrointestinal Tract Oncogenesis. *Metabolism* **2018**, *87*, 18–24. [CrossRef] [PubMed]
13. Feilstrecker Balani, G.; Dos Santos Cortez, M.; Picasky da Silveira Freitas, J.E.; Freire de Melo, F.; Zarpelon-Schutz, A.C.; Teixeira K.N. Immune Response Modulation in Inflammatory Bowel Diseases by Helicobacter Pylori Infection. *World J. Gastroenterol.* **2023**, *29*, 4604–4615. [CrossRef] [PubMed]
14. Sulaiman, C.T.; Anju, K.A.; Anandan, E.; Balachandran, I. Synergistic Interactions of Phytochemicals in Polyherbal Formulation Enhance the Chemical Transformations of Active Constituents. *J. Appl. Spectrosc.* **2021**, *88*, 181–186. [CrossRef]
15. Mattioli, L.B.; Frosini, M.; Corazza, I.; Fiorino, S.; Zippi, M.; Micucci, M.; Budriesi, R. Long COVID-19 Gastrointestinal Related Disorders and Traditional Chinese Medicine: A Network Target-Based Approach. *Phytother. Res.* **2024**, *38*, 2323–2346. [CrossRef]
16. Mobeen, A.; Moazzam, S.W. Jawarish Shahi: A Special Dosage Form of Herbal Formulations for Functional Gastrointestinal Disorders in Unani Medicine—A Comprehensive Review. *J. Ethnopharmacol.* **2022**, *293*, 115319. [CrossRef]
17. Dubey, R.K.; Shukla, S. Exploring Novel Herbal Compounds and Formulations for Inflammatory Bowel Disease (IBD) Management. *Zhongguo Ying Yong Sheng Li Xue Za Zhi* **2023**, *39*, e20230003. [CrossRef]
18. Lashgari, N.-A.; Roudsari, N.M.; Momtaz, S.; Niazi Shahraki, F.; Zandi, N.; Pazoki, B.; Farzaei, M.H.; Ghasemi, M.; Abdollahi M.; Abdolghaffari, A.H. Systematic Review on Herbal Preparations for Controlling Visceral Hypersensitivity in Functional Gastrointestinal Disorders. *Curr. Pharm. Biotechnol.* **2024**, *25*, 1632–1650. [CrossRef]
19. Singh, R.; Zogg, H.; Ghoshal, U.C.; Ro, S. Current Treatment Options and Therapeutic Insights for Gastrointestinal Dysmotility and Functional Gastrointestinal Disorders. *Front. Pharmacol.* **2022**, *13*, 808195. [CrossRef]
20. Zhang, R.; Zhu, X.; Bai, H.; Ning, K. Network Pharmacology Databases for Traditional Chinese Medicine: Review and Assessment *Front. Pharmacol.* **2019**, *10*, 123. [CrossRef]
21. Narayanan, A.S.; Raja, S.S.S.; Ponmurugan, K.; Kandekar, S.C.; Natarajaseenivasan, K.; Maripandi, A.; Mandeel, Q.A. Antibacterial Activity of Selected Medicinal Plants against Multiple Antibiotic Resistant Uropathogens: A Study from Kolli Hills, Tamil Nadu, India. *Benef. Microbes* **2011**, *2*, 235–243. [CrossRef] [PubMed]
22. Bopana, N.; Saxena, S. Asparagus Racemosus--Ethnopharmacological Evaluation and Conservation Needs. *J. Ethnopharmacol.* **2007**, *110*, 1–15. [CrossRef] [PubMed]
23. Mandal, S.C.; Nandy, A.; Pal, M.; Saha, B.P. Evaluation of Antibacterial Activity of Asparagus Racemosus Willd. Root. *Phytother. Res.* **2000**, *14*, 118–119. [CrossRef]
24. Datta, G.K.; Sairam, K.; Priyambada, S.; Debnath, P.K.; Goel, R.K. Antiulcerogenic Activity of Satavari Mandur--an Ayurvedic Herbo-Mineral Preparation. *Indian. J. Exp. Biol.* **2002**, *40*, 1173–1177.
25. Bhatnagar, M.; Sisodia, S.S. Antisecretory and Antiulcer Activity of Asparagus Racemosus Willd. against Indomethacin plus Phyloric Ligation-Induced Gastric Ulcer in Rats. *J. Herb. Pharmacother.* **2006**, *6*, 13–20. [CrossRef]
26. Bhatnagar, M.; Sisodia, S.S.; Bhatnagar, R. Antiulcer and Antioxidant Activity of Asparagus Racemosus Willd and Withania Somnifera Dunal in Rats. *Ann. N. Y. Acad. Sci.* **2005**, *1056*, 261–278. [CrossRef]
27. Venkatesan, N.; Thiyagarajan, V.; Narayanan, S.; Arul, A.; Raja, S.; Vijaya Kumar, S.G.; Rajarajan, T.; Perianayagam, J.B. Anti-Diarrhoeal Potential of Asparagus Racemosus Wild Root Extracts in Laboratory Animals. *J. Pharm. Pharm. Sci.* **2005**, *8*, 39–46.
28. Twardowschy, A.; Freitas, C.S.; Baggio, C.H.; Mayer, B.; dos Santos, A.C.; Pizzolatti, M.G.; Zacarias, A.A.; dos Santos, E.P.; Otuki, M.F.; Marques, M.C.A. Antiulcerogenic Activity of Bark Extract of Tabebuia Avellanedae, Lorentz Ex Griseb. *J. Ethnopharmacol.* **2008**, *118*, 455–459. [CrossRef]
29. Goel, R.K.; Pathak, N.K.; Biswas, M.; Pandey, V.B.; Sanyal, A.K. Effect of Lapachol, a Naphthaquinone Isolated from Tectona Grandis, on Experimental Peptic Ulcer and Gastric Secretion. *J. Pharm. Pharmacol.* **1987**, *39*, 138–140. [CrossRef]
30. van Uum, S.H. Liquorice and Hypertension. *Neth. J. Med.* **2005**, *63*, 119–120.
31. Chen, G.; Zhu, L.; Liu, Y.; Zhou, Q.; Chen, H.; Yang, J. Isoliquiritigenin, a Flavonoid from Licorice, Plays a Dual Role in Regulating Gastrointestinal Motility in Vitro and in Vivo. *Phytother. Res.* **2009**, *23*, 498–506. [CrossRef] [PubMed]
32. Zhang, D.; Gan, R.-Y.; Zhang, J.-R.; Farha, A.K.; Li, H.-B.; Zhu, F.; Wang, X.-H.; Corke, H. Antivirulence Properties and Related Mechanisms of Spice Essential Oils: A Comprehensive Review. *Compr. Rev. Food Sci. Food Saf.* **2020**, *19*, 1018–1055. [CrossRef] [PubMed]
33. Thapa, D.; Losa, R.; Zweifel, B.; Wallace, R.J. Sensitivity of Pathogenic and Commensal Bacteria from the Human Colon to Essential Oils. *Microbiology* **2012**, *158*, 2870–2877. [CrossRef] [PubMed]
34. Badgujar, S.B.; Patel, V.V.; Bandivdekar, A.H. Foeniculum Vulgare Mill: A Review of Its Botany, Phytochemistry, Pharmacology, Contemporary Application, and Toxicology. *Biomed. Res. Int.* **2014**, *2014*, 842674. [CrossRef] [PubMed]
35. Brković, D.L.; Čomić, L.; Solujić, S.S. Antibacterial Activity of Some Plants from Family Apiaceae in Relation to Selected Phytopathogenic Bacteria. *Kragujev. J. Sci.* **2006**, *28*, 65–72.
36. Gulfraz, M.; Mehmood, S.; Minhas, N.; Jabeen, N.; Kausar, R.; Jabeen, K.; Arshad, G. Composition and Antimicrobial Properties of Essential Oil of Foeniculum Vulgare. *Afr. J. Biotechnol.* **2008**, *7*, 4364–4368.
37. Ozbek, H.; Uğraş, S.; Dülger, H.; Bayram, I.; Tuncer, I.; Oztürk, G.; Oztürk, A. Hepatoprotective Effect of Foeniculum Vulgare Essential Oil. *Fitoterapia* **2003**, *74*, 317–319. [CrossRef]

38. Asano, T.; Aida, S.; Suemasu, S.; Mizushima, T. Anethole Restores Delayed Gastric Emptying and Impaired Gastric Accommodation in Rodents. *Biochem. Biophys. Res. Commun.* **2016**, *472*, 125–130. [CrossRef]
39. Carrillo, E.; Ramírez-Rivera, S.; Bernal, G.; Aquea, G.; Tessini, C.; Thomet, F.A. Water-Soluble Ru(II)-Anethole Compounds with Promising Cytotoxicity toward the Human Gastric Cancer Cell Line AGS. *Life Sci.* **2019**, *217*, 193–201. [CrossRef]
40. Zhao, H.; Ren, S.; Yang, H.; Tang, S.; Guo, C.; Liu, M.; Tao, Q.; Ming, T.; Xu, H. Peppermint Essential Oil: Its Phytochemistry, Biological Activity, Pharmacological Effect and Application. *Biomed. Pharmacother.* **2022**, *154*, 113559. [CrossRef]
41. Acker, B.W.; Cash, B.D. Medicinal Foods for Functional GI Disorders. *Curr. Gastroenterol. Rep.* **2017**, *19*, 62. [CrossRef] [PubMed]
42. Dumitrescu, E.; Muselin, F.; Tîrziu, E.; Folescu, M.; Dumitrescu, C.S.; Orboi, D.M.; Cristina, R.T. *Pimpinella Anisum* L. Essential Oil a Valuable Antibacterial and Antifungal Alternative. *Plants* **2023**, *12*, 2428. [CrossRef] [PubMed]
43. Wang, Y.; Minden, A. Current Molecular Combination Therapies Used for the Treatment of Breast Cancer. *Int. J. Mol. Sci.* **2022**, *23*, 11046. [CrossRef] [PubMed]
44. Mattioli, L.B.; Corazza, I.; Budriesi, R.; Hrelia, S.; Malaguti, M.; Caliceti, C.; Amoroso, R.; Maccallini, C.; Crupi, P.; Clodoveo, M.L.; et al. From Waste to Health: Olive Mill Wastewater for Cardiovascular Disease Prevention. *Nutrients* **2024**, *16*, 2986. [CrossRef]
45. Cavalluzzi, M.M.; Lamonaca, A.; Rotondo, N.P.; Miniero, D.V.; Muraglia, M.; Gabriele, P.; Corbo, F.; De Palma, A.; Budriesi, R.; De Angelis, E.; et al. Microwave-Assisted Extraction of Bioactive Compounds from Lentil Wastes: Antioxidant Activity Evaluation and Metabolomic Characterization. *Molecules* **2022**, *27*, 7471. [CrossRef]
46. Micucci, M.; Angeletti, A.; Cont, M.; Corazza, I.; Aldini, R.; Donadio, E.; Chiarini, A.; Budriesi, R. *Hibiscus Sabdariffa* L. Flowers and *Olea Europea* L. Leaves Extract-Based Formulation for Hypertension Care: In Vitro Efficacy and Toxicological Profile. *J. Med. Food* **2016**, *19*, 504–512. [CrossRef]
47. Roselli, M.; Carocci, A.; Budriesi, R.; Micucci, M.; Toma, M.; Di Cesare Mannelli, L.; Lovece, A.; Catalano, A.; Cavalluzzi, M.M.; Bruno, C.; et al. Synthesis, Antiarrhythmic Activity, and Toxicological Evaluation of Mexiletine Analogues. *Eur. J. Med. Chem.* **2016**, *121*, 300–307. [CrossRef]
48. Milani, G.; Budriesi, R.; Tavazzani, E.; Cavalluzzi, M.M.; Mattioli, L.B.; Miniero, D.V.; Delre, P.; Belviso, B.D.; Denegri, M.; Cuocci, C.; et al. hERG Stereoselective Modulation by Mexiletine-Derived Ureas: Molecular Docking Study, Synthesis, and Biological Evaluation. *Arch. Pharm.* **2023**, *356*, e2300116. [CrossRef]
49. Mattioli, L.B.; Frosini, M.; Amoroso, R.; Maccallini, C.; Chiano, E.; Aldini, R.; Urso, F.; Corazza, I.; Micucci, M.; Budriesi, R. *Olea Europea* L. Leaves and *Hibiscus Sabdariffa* L. Petals Extracts: Herbal Mix from Cardiovascular Network Target to Gut Motility Dysfunction Application. *Nutrients* **2022**, *14*, 463. [CrossRef]
50. Saheera, S.; Potnuri, A.G.; Guha, A.; Palaniyandi, S.S.; Thandavarayan, R.A. Histamine 2 Receptors in Cardiovascular Biology: A Friend for the Heart. *Drug Discov. Today* **2022**, *27*, 234–245. [CrossRef]
51. Tallarida, R.J.; Murray, R.B. Mean, Standard Deviation, and Confidence Limits. In *Manual of Pharmacologic Calculations: With Computer Programs*; Tallarida, R.J., Murray, R.B., Eds.; Springer: New York, NY, USA, 1987; pp. 7–10. ISBN 978-1-4612-4974-0.
52. Motulsky, H.; Christopoulos, A. *Fitting Models to Biological Data Using Linear and Nonlinear Regression: A Practical Guide to Curve Fitting*; Oxford University Press: New York, NY, USA, 2004; ISBN 978-0-19-517179-2.
53. Motulsky, H.J. *Prism 5 Statistics Guide*; GraphPad Software Inc.: San Diego, CA, USA, 2007.
54. Balouiri, M.; Sadiki, M.; Ibnsouda, S.K. Methods for *in Vitro* Evaluating Antimicrobial Activity: A Review. *J. Pharm. Anal.* **2016**, *6*, 71–79. [CrossRef] [PubMed]
55. Benzie, I.F.F.; Strain, J.J. The Ferric Reducing Ability of Plasma (FRAP) as a Measure of "Antioxidant Power": The FRAP Assay. *Anal. Biochem.* **1996**, *239*, 70–76. [CrossRef] [PubMed]
56. Orav, A.; Raal, A.; Arak, E. Essential Oil Composition of *Pimpinella Anisum* L. Fruits from Various European Countries. *Nat. Prod. Res.* **2008**, *22*, 227–232. [CrossRef] [PubMed]
57. Raal, A.; Orav, A.; Arak, E. Essential Oil Composition of Foeniculum Vulgare Mill. Fruits from Pharmacies in Different Countries. *Nat. Prod. Res.* **2012**, *26*, 1173–1178. [CrossRef]
58. Basaglia, G.; Fiori, J.; Leoni, A.; Gotti, R. Determination of Estragole in Fennel Herbal Teas by HS-SPME and GC–MS. *Anal. Lett.* **2014**, *47*, 368–379. [CrossRef]
59. Fiori, J.; Naldi, M.; Gotti, R. HS–SPME–GC–MS for the Quantitation and Chiral Characterization of Camphor and Menthol in Creams. *Chromatographia* **2010**, *72*, 941–947. [CrossRef]
60. Curci, F.; Corbo, F.; Clodoveo, M.L.; Salvagno, L.; Rosato, A.; Corazza, I.; Budriesi, R.; Micucci, M.; Mattioli, L.B. Polyphenols from Olive-Mill Wastewater and Biological Activity: Focus on Irritable Bowel Syndrome. *Nutrients* **2022**, *14*, 1264. [CrossRef]
61. Chiarini, A.; Minarini, A.; Budriesi, R.; Melchiorre, C. Molecular Properties of the Histamine H2-Receptor. Covalent Inhibition by Tetraamine Disulfides. *Farmaco* **1990**, *45*, 1001–1011.
62. Hajimahmoodi, M.; Shams-Ardakani, M.; Saniee, P.; Siavoshi, F.; Mehrabani, M.; Hosseinzadeh, H.; Foroumadi, P.; Safavi, M.; Khanavi, M.; Akbarzadeh, T.; et al. In Vitro Antibacterial Activity of Some Iranian Medicinal Plant Extracts against Helicobacter Pylori. *Nat. Prod. Res.* **2011**, *25*, 1059–1066. [CrossRef]
63. Tabak, M.; Armon, R.; Neeman, I. Cinnamon Extracts' Inhibitory Effect on *Helicobacter Pylori*. *J. Ethnopharmacol.* **1999**, *67*, 269–277. [CrossRef]
64. Masadeh, M.M.; Alkofahi, A.S.; Alzoubi, K.H.; Tumah, H.N.; Bani-Hani, K. Anti-Helicobactor Pylori Activity of Some Jordanian Medicinal Plants. *Pharm. Biol.* **2014**, *52*, 566–569. [CrossRef] [PubMed]

65. Ngnameko, C.R.; Marchetti, L.; Zambelli, B.; Quotadamo, A.; Roncarati, D.; Bertelli, D.; Njayou, F.N.; Smith, S.I.; Moundipa, P.F.; Costi, M.P.; et al. New Insights into Bioactive Compounds from the Medicinal Plant Spathodea Campanulata P. Beauv. and Their Activity against Helicobacter Pylori. *Antibiotics* **2020**, *9*, 258. [CrossRef] [PubMed]
66. Fukai, T.; Marumo, A.; Kaitou, K.; Kanda, T.; Terada, S.; Nomura, T. Anti-*Helicobacter Pylori* Flavonoids from Licorice Extract. *Life Sci.* **2002**, *71*, 1449–1463. [CrossRef] [PubMed]
67. Kusano, M.; Hosaka, H.; Kawada, A.; Kuribayashi, S.; Shimoyama, Y.; Zai, H.; Kawamura, O.; Yamada, M. Gastrointestinal Motility and Functional Gastrointestinal Diseases. *Curr. Pharm. Des.* **2014**, *20*, 2775–2782. [CrossRef]
68. Sanders, K.M.; Koh, S.D.; Ro, S.; Ward, S.M. Regulation of Gastrointestinal Motility—Insights from Smooth Muscle Biology. *Nat. Rev. Gastroenterol. Hepatol.* **2012**, *9*, 633–645. [CrossRef]
69. Hildebrand, F.; Ebersbach, T.; Nielsen, H.B.; Li, X.; Sonne, S.B.; Bertalan, M.; Dimitrov, P.; Madsen, L.; Qin, J.; Wang, J.; et al. A Comparative Analysis of the Intestinal Metagenomes Present in Guinea Pigs (*Cavia porcellus*) and Humans (*Homo sapiens*). *BMC Genom.* **2012**, *13*, 514. [CrossRef]
70. Poitras, P.; Honde, C.; Havrankova, J.; Lahaie, R.G.; Trudel, L.; Goyer, R.; Junien, J.L.; Pascaud, X. Effect of Trimebutine on Intestinal Motility and Plasma Motilin in the Dog. *Am. J. Physiol.* **1986**, *251*, G349–G353. [CrossRef]
71. Carocci, A.; Roselli, M.; Budriesi, R.; Micucci, M.; Desaphy, J.-F.; Altamura, C.; Cavalluzzi, M.M.; Toma, M.; Passeri, G.I.; Milani, G.; et al. Synthesis and Evaluation of Voltage-Gated Sodium Channel Blocking Pyrroline Derivatives Endowed with Both Antiarrhythmic and Antioxidant Activities. *ChemMedChem* **2021**, *16*, 578–588. [CrossRef]
72. Ioan, P.; Carosati, E.; Micucci, M.; Cruciani, G.; Broccatelli, F.; Zhorov, B.S.; Chiarini, A.; Budriesi, R. 1,4-Dihydropyridine Scaffold in Medicinal Chemistry, the Story so Far and Perspectives (Part 1): Action in Ion Channels and GPCRs. *Curr. Med. Chem.* **2011**, *18*, 4901–4922. [CrossRef]
73. Evangelista, S. Otilonium Bromide: A Selective Spasmolytic for the Gastrointestinal Tract. *J. Int. Med. Res.* **1999**, *27*, 207–222. [CrossRef]
74. Strege, P.R.; Evangelista, S.; Lyford, G.L.; Sarr, M.G.; Farrugia, G. Otilonium Bromide Inhibits Calcium Entry through L-Type Calcium Channels in Human Intestinal Smooth Muscle. *Neurogastroenterol. Motil.* **2004**, *16*, 167–173. [CrossRef] [PubMed]
75. Boeckxstaens, G.; Corazziari, E.S.; Mearin, F.; Tack, J. IBS and the Role of Otilonium Bromide. *Int. J. Colorectal Dis.* **2013**, *28*, 295–304. [CrossRef] [PubMed]
76. Korecka, A.; Arulampalam, V. The Gut Microbiome: Scourge, Sentinel or Spectator? *J. Oral. Microbiol.* **2012**, *4*, 9367. [CrossRef] [PubMed]
77. Martinsen, T.C.; Bergh, K.; Waldum, H.L. Gastric Juice: A Barrier against Infectious Diseases. *Basic. Clin. Pharmacol. Toxicol.* **2005**, *96*, 94–102. [CrossRef]
78. Naylor, G.; Axon, A. Role of Bacterial Overgrowth in the Stomach as an Additional Risk Factor for Gastritis. *Can. J. Gastroenterol.* **2003**, *17* (Suppl. B), 13B–17B. [CrossRef]
79. Reyes, V.E. Helicobacter Pylori and Its Role in Gastric Cancer. *Microorganisms* **2023**, *11*, 1312. [CrossRef]
80. Huang, J.; Sridhar, S.; Hunt, R. Role of Helicobacter Pylori Infection and Non-Steroidal Anti-Inflammatory Drugs in Peptic-Ulcer Disease: A Meta-Analysis. *Lancet* **2002**, *359*, 14–22. [CrossRef]
81. Park, Y.H.; Kim, N. Review of Atrophic Gastritis and Intestinal Metaplasia as a Premalignant Lesion of Gastric Cancer. *J. Cancer Prev.* **2015**, *20*, 25–40. [CrossRef]
82. Yang, J.-C.; Lu, C.-W.; Lin, C.-J. Treatment of Helicobacter Pylori Infection: Current Status and Future Concepts. *World J. Gastroenterol.* **2014**, *20*, 5283–5293. [CrossRef]
83. Nostro, A.; Cellini, L.; Di Bartolomeo, S.; Di Campli, E.; Grande, R.; Cannatelli, M.A.; Marzio, L.; Alonzo, V. Antibacterial Effect of Plant Extracts against Helicobacter Pylori. *Phytother. Res.* **2005**, *19*, 198–202. [CrossRef]
84. Imai, H.; Osawa, K.; Yasuda, H.; Hamashima, H.; Arai, T.; Sasatsu, M. Inhibition by the Essential Oils of Peppermint and Spearmint of the Growth of Pathogenic Bacteria. *Microbios* **2001**, *106* (Suppl. 1), 31–39. [PubMed]
85. Marwa, C.; Fikri-Benbrahim, K.; Ou-Yahia, D.; Farah, A. African Peppermint (Mentha Piperita) from Morocco: Chemical Composition and Antimicrobial Properties of Essential Oil. *J. Adv. Pharm. Technol. Res.* **2017**, *8*, 86–90. [CrossRef] [PubMed]
86. Alomar, H.A.; Fathallah, N.; Abdel-Aziz, M.M.; Ibrahim, T.A.; Elkady, W.M. GC-MS Profiling, Anti-Helicobacter Pylori, and Anti-Inflammatory Activities of Three Apiaceous Fruits' Essential Oils. *Plants* **2022**, *11*, 2617. [CrossRef] [PubMed]
87. Sathianarayanan, S.; Ammanath, A.V.; Biswas, R.; Anita, B.; Sukumaran, S.; Venkidasamy, B. A New Approach against Helicobacter Pylori Using Plants and Its Constituents: A Review Study. *Microb. Pathog.* **2022**, *168*, 105594. [CrossRef]
88. Nazari, S.; Rameshrad, M.; Hosseinzadeh, H. Toxicological Effects of Glycyrrhiza Glabra (Licorice): A Review. *Phytother. Res.* **2017**, *31*, 1635–1650. [CrossRef]
89. Wahab, S.; Annadurai, S.; Abullais, S.S.; Das, G.; Ahmad, W.; Ahmad, M.F.; Kandasamy, G.; Vasudevan, R.; Ali, M.S.; Amir, M. Glycyrrhiza Glabra (Licorice): A Comprehensive Review on Its Phytochemistry, Biological Activities, Clinical Evidence and Toxicology. *Plants* **2021**, *10*, 2751. [CrossRef]
90. do Nascimento, M.H.M.; de Araújo, D.R. Exploring the Pharmacological Potential of Glycyrrhizic Acid: From Therapeutic Applications to Trends in Nanomedicine. *Future Pharmacol.* **2022**, *2*, 1–15. [CrossRef]
91. Li, B.; Cheung, K.S.; Wong, I.Y.-H.; Leung, W.K.; Law, S. Calcium Channel Blockers Are Associated with Lower Gastric Cancer Risk: A Territory-Wide Study with Propensity Score Analysis. *Int. J. Cancer* **2021**, *148*, 2148–2157. [CrossRef]

92. Carosati, E.; Ioan, P.; Micucci, M.; Broccatelli, F.; Cruciani, G.; Zhorov, B.S.; Chiarini, A.; Budriesi, R. 1,4-Dihydropyridine Scaffold in Medicinal Chemistry, The Story So Far And Perspectives (Part 2): Action in Other Targets and Antitargets. *Curr. Med. Chem.* **2012**, *19*, 4306–4323. [CrossRef]
93. Salem, M.S.E.-D.; Mahfouz, A.Y.; Fathy, R.M. The Antibacterial and Antihemolytic Activities Assessment of Zinc Oxide Nanoparticles Synthesized Using Plant Extracts and Gamma Irradiation against the Uro-Pathogenic Multidrug Resistant Proteus Vulgaris. *Biometals* **2021**, *34*, 175–196. [CrossRef]
94. Onlom, C.; Khanthawong, S.; Waranuch, N.; Ingkaninan, K. In vitro anti-Malassezia activity and potential use in anti-dandruff formulation of Asparagus racemosus. *Int. J. Cosmet. Sci.* **2014**, *36*, 74–78. [CrossRef] [PubMed]
95. Shaha, P.; Bellankimath, A. Pharmacological Profile of Asparagus Racemosus: A Review. *Int. J. Curr. Microbiol. Appl. Sci.* **2017**, *6*, 1215–1223. [CrossRef]
96. Singh, R. Asparagus Racemosus: A Review on Its Phytochemical and Therapeutic Potential. *Nat. Prod. Res.* **2016**, *30*, 1896–1908. [CrossRef] [PubMed]
97. Chakŭrski, I.; Matev, M.; Koĭchev, A.; Angelova, I.; Stefanov, G. Treatment of chronic colitis with an herbal combination of Taraxacum officinale, Hipericum perforatum, Melissa officinaliss, Calendula officinalis and Foeniculum vulgare. *Vutr. Boles.* **1981**, *20*, 51–54.
98. Pradhan, M.; Sribhuwaneswari, S.; Karthikeyan, D.; Minz, S.; Sure, P.; Chandu, A.N.; Mishra, U.; Kamalakannan, K.; Saravanakumar, A.; Sivakumar, T. In-Vitro Cytoprotection Activity of Foeniculum Vulgare and Helicteres Isora in Cultured Human Blood Lymphocytes and Antitumour Activity against B16F10 Melanoma Cell Line. *Res. J. Pharm. Technol.* **2008**, *1*, 450–452.
99. Tabebuia—An Overview | ScienceDirect Topics. Available online: https://www.sciencedirect.com/topics/pharmacology-toxicology-and-pharmaceutical-science/tabebuia (accessed on 30 October 2024).
100. Kalpoutzakis, E.; Chatzimitakos, T.; Athanasiadis, V.; Mitakou, S.; Aligiannis, N.; Bozinou, E.; Gortzi, O.; Skaltsounis, L.A.; Lalas, S.I. Determination of the Total Phenolics Content and Antioxidant Activity of Extracts from Parts of Plants from the Greek Island of Crete. *Plants* **2023**, *12*, 1092. [CrossRef]
101. Tovar, R.T.; Petzel, R.M. Herbal Toxicity. *Dis. Mon.* **2009**, *55*, 592–641. [CrossRef]
102. Heinrich, M. Quality and Safety of Herbal Medical Products: Regulation and the Need for Quality Assurance along the Value Chains. *Br. J. Clin. Pharmacol.* **2015**, *80*, 62–66. [CrossRef]
103. Farrar, A.J.; Farrar, F.C. Clinical Aromatherapy. *Nurs. Clin. North. Am.* **2020**, *55*, 489–504. [CrossRef]
104. Drossman, D.A. Functional Gastrointestinal Disorders: History, Pathophysiology, Clinical Features and Rome IV. *Gastroenterology* **2016**, *150*, 1262–1279.e2. [CrossRef]
105. Leri, M.; Scuto, M.; Ontario, M.L.; Calabrese, V.; Calabrese, E.J.; Bucciantini, M.; Stefani, M. Healthy Effects of Plant Polyphenols: Molecular Mechanisms. *Int. J. Mol. Sci.* **2020**, *21*, 1250. [CrossRef]
106. Roe, A.L.; Paine, M.F.; Gurley, B.J.; Brouwer, K.R.; Jordan, S.; Griffiths, J.C. Assessing Natural Product-Drug Interactions: An End-to-End Safety Framework. *Regul. Toxicol. Pharmacol.* **2016**, *76*, 1–6. [CrossRef]

nutrients

MDPI

Article

The Effect of Flavonoids and Topiramate on Glucose Carbon Metabolism in a HepG2 Steatosis Cell Culture Model: A Stable Isotope Study

Li Ma [1,2], Qing-Yi Lu [3], Shu Lim [1], Guang Han [1], Laszlo G. Boros [4], Mina Desai [1,5] and Jennifer K. Yee [1,6,*]

1 The Lundquist Institute of Biomedical Innovation at Harbor-UCLA Medical Center, 1124 West Carson Street, Torrance, CA 90502, USA; mariecurie@126.com (L.M.); ghan@lundquist.org (G.H.); mdesai@lundquiast.org (M.D.)

2 Jiangsu Key Laboratory for the Research and Utilization of Plant Resources, Institute of Botany, Jiangsu Province and Chinese Academy of Sciences (Nanjing Botanical Garden Memorial Sun Yat-Sen), No. 1 Qianhuhoucun Village, Zhongshan Gate, Nanjing 210014, China

3 Center for Human Nutrition, Department of Medicine, and Department of Pathology and Laboratory Medicine, David Geffen School of Medicine at the University of California, 10833 Le Conte Avenue, Los Angeles, CA 90095, USA

4 Medicine and Health Care Division, Hungarian Society of Natural Sciences, Jászai Mari Square 4/a, Floor/Door 1/1, H-1137 Budapest, Hungary; contact@laszlogboros.com

5 Department of Obstetrics and Gynecology, David Geffen School of Medicine at the University of California, Los Angeles, 10833 Le Conte Avenue, Los Angeles, CA 90095, USA

6 Department of Pediatrics, David Geffen School of Medicine at the University of California, 10833 Le Conte Avenue, Los Angeles, CA 90095, USA

* Correspondence: jyee@lundquist.org; Tel.: +1-310-222-8175

Abstract: Background: Insufficient treatment options are available for metabolic dysfunction-associated steatotic liver disease (MASLD). Flavonoids and topiramate have been studied for weight loss but need investigation into their effects on liver metabolism. This study's aim was to examine the effects of flavonoids or topiramate on glucose metabolic carbon flux in a cell culture model of steatosis. **Methods**: Steatosis was induced in HepG2 cells through exposure to oleic acid (OA, 0.5 mml/L) conjugated to bovine serum albumin (2:1). Additionally, 50% U^{13}C-glucose was supplied in the medium as a stable isotope tracer. Cells were treated with DMSO, 10 μM of naringenin, morin, silibinin, or topiramate (44 μM) for 72 h. A non-steatotic, untreated HepG2 cell control was included. Cell extracts were analyzed by gas chromatography/mass spectrometry and mass isotopomer distribution analysis for glycogen synthesis, de novo fatty acid synthesis, tricarboxylic acid (TCA) cycle activity, and ribose synthesis. Groups were compared by ANOVA with Tukey's pair-wise testing. **Results**: Compared to untreated HepG2 controls, OA-exposed steatotic cells exhibited increased lipid accumulation by ORO staining (1.6-fold), enhanced palmitate de novo synthesis, reduced pyruvate carboxylase/pyruvate dehydrogenase (PC/PDH) ratio, and reduced ribose synthesis. Treatment with topiramate or silibinin ameliorated the lipid accumulation (1.3-fold) and mitigated enhancement of de novo synthesis. Morin-treated cells exhibited enhanced de novo synthesis but suppressed ribose synthesis. **Conclusions**: Potential mechanisms of reduced lipid accumulation by topiramate and silibinin may include suppression of palmitate de novo synthesis and a relative decrease in carbon flux through the PDH pathway. Further studies are needed on potential utility in MASLD based on their specific metabolic effects.

Keywords: hepatic steatosis; flavonoid; stable isotope; lipid; carbon flux

https://doi.org/10.3390/nu17030564

1. Introduction

The condition previously known as non-alcoholic fatty liver disease (NAFLD) affects up to 30% of the US population [1]. Now redefined as metabolic dysfunction-associated steatotic liver disease, MASLD ranges from simple steatosis that may progress over time to metabolic dysfunction-associated steatohepatitis (MASH) with inflammation and fibrosis. The enhanced lipid accumulation in hepatocytes increases susceptibility to oxidative stress, proinflammatory cytokines, and cell death. Eventually, MASH may further progress to cirrhosis and finally hepatocellular carcinoma [2]. In addition to the liver-related morbidity and mortality, MASLD is associated with cardiovascular disease as well as T2DM, cancer, and chronic kidney disease.

Current treatment options are lacking. There is only one Food and Drug Administration-approved treatment for MASH, but no approved pharmacologic agents for earlier stages of MASLD to prevent MASH. Healthy nutrition and increased physical activity to promote weight loss remain the cornerstones of management of MASLD. In clinical care, individuals with MASLD are advised to consume a diet low in refined carbohydrates and saturated fats to reduce liver lipid production and accumulation. They are recommended to eat more fruits, vegetables, fish, and whole grains, which include antioxidant nutrients that may decrease cellular stress and inflammation. Specific foods and dietary patterns appear to be associated with better outcomes related to MASLD from systematic reviews and/or meta-analyses (SRMA). One publication that included eleven observational studies showed lower risk of MASLD among people with higher fruit and vegetable intake [3]. Another SRMA that incorporated data from nine studies demonstrated an association between coffee consumption and reduced liver fibrosis, although the general incidence of MASLD was not different [4]. Another meta-analysis that included data from four clinical trials showed improved liver function tests with green tea supplementation [5]. Therefore, research on interventions for MASLD includes the search for potential bioactive molecules found in these foods that might confer hepatoprotective effects.

Coffee, tea, and berries are food sources high in flavonoids, and these compounds have garnered much interest for their potential roles in modulating MASLD. Naringenin, derived from citrus fruit, has been shown in a number of in vitro and animal studies to modulate several biological processes implicated in MASLD, including increasing expression of peroxisome proliferator-activated receptor (PPAR)α and PPARγ and other downstream targets, regulating energy balance, improving fatty acid oxidation, modulating lipid metabolism, and reducing liver triglyceride accumulation, oxidative stress, and inflammation [6]. Silibinin, from extract of milk thistle, may antagonize the progression of MASLD by intervening in oxidative stress, insulin resistance, liver fat accumulation, and mitochondrial dysfunction [7]. A multicenter, phase III, double-blind clinical trial on 180 patients with histological diagnosis of NAFLD/NASH with or without hepatitis C demonstrated that treatment with a silybin–vitamin E–phosphatidylcholine complex for 12 months supported improvement of transaminase and γ-GT levels, along with improvement of insulin sensitivity. In 35 treated patients, a clear improvement of steatosis, lobular inflammation, ballooning, and liver fibrosis was observed compared to baseline [8]. Morin, a flavonol from mulberry and other plants, has alleviated the development of MASLD in high-fat-diet-induced obese mice, reduced body weight gain and triglyceride levels, and improved glucose tolerance, mediated by the suppression of liver X receptor (LXR) signaling [9]. Another study reported that morin mitigates reactive tumor necrosis factor-α (TNF-α) level and triglyceride accumulation in OA-induced HepG2 cells and in tyloxapol-induced mice through upregulation of PPARα and suppression of sterol regulatory element-binding protein 1c (SREBP-1c) [10]. In general, these dietary flavonoids are potent antioxidants and exhibit anti-inflammatory, antifibrotic, and antihyperglycemic effects, and therefore are potentially protective against MASLD [6,11,12].

Topiramate is an FDA-approved medication for treating epilepsy and migraines and promoting weight loss in combination with phentermine. Topiramate has a variety of physiologic effects including neurotransmitter effects through promotion of activity of the gamma-amino butyric acid (GABA)-A receptor, inhibition of glutamate receptor, and inhibition of carbonic anhydrase. Human studies have reported positively on the weight-loss-promoting and insulin-sensitizing properties of topiramate [13–15], in addition to improvements in circulating lipid levels. One rare case report suggested a potential role in improvement of MASLD after an adolescent lost significant body weight on topiramate and also experienced improvement in liver enzymes and hepatic steatosis. In Wistar rats fed a high-fat/high-fructose diet to induce insulin resistance with elevated ALT and glucose intolerance, animals treated with topiramate exhibited normal glucose tolerance, improvement of ALT, and increased adiponectin levels [16]. However, the study did not specifically address MASLD. Therefore, more data are needed regarding potential direct effects of topiramate on liver metabolic pathways as a potential treatment for MASLD.

Tracer-based metabolomics provides a highly comprehensive yet specific architecture to examine relationships among multiple pathways in living systems. Earlier studies using gas chromatography/mass spectrometry (GC/MS) have previously demonstrated the utility of this approach as a systems biology tool to identify perturbations of cellular metabolic pathways in response to the treatment of plant-derived bioactive small molecules [17–19]. Metabolites that incorporate stable isotope tracers therefore represent dynamic functional outcomes [20]. Glucose has implications in MASLD from the nutrient standpoint, serving as a substrate that donates its carbons toward multiple interconnected metabolic pathways, including glycogen synthesis, nucleotide synthesis, and lipogenesis. Therefore, use of ^{13}C as a stable isotope tracer provides an opportunity to observe perturbations in the liver metabolic network over the course of an intervention. The aim of the present study was to determine the effects of three flavonoids, naringenin, morin, silibinin, and the weight-loss promoting drug topiramate on glucose-derived carbon flux in steatotic liver cell culture using $U^{13}C$-glucose as a stable isotope tracer. We hypothesized that these compounds might promote relative pathway activities in favor of decreased liver steatosis, possibly through decreasing glucose utilization toward liver lipogenesis.

2. Materials and Methods

2.1. Chemicals

Morin (2-(2,4-dihydroxyphenyl)-3,5,7-trihydroxychromen-4-one), naringenin (5,7-dihydroxy-2-(4-hydroxyphenyl)chroman-4-one), silibinin (2,3-dihydro-3-(4-hydroxy-3-methoxyphenyl)-2-(hydroxymethyl)-6-(3,5,7-trihydroxy-4-oxobenz opyran-2-yl)benzodioxin), topiramate, glucose, and Oil Red O staining kit were purchased from Sigma-Aldrich (St. Louis, MO, USA). Naringenin and morin were also purchased from Chengdu Mansite Pharmaceutical Co, LTD (Chengdu, China). [$U^{13}C6$]-D-glucose isotope was purchased from Cambridge Isotope Laboratories (Tewksbury, MA, USA) with 99% purity and 99% isotope enrichment for each position. Cell Counting Kit-8 assay kit, total protein assay kit (with standard: BCA method), Antibodies for Western blotting (FAS, SREBP1, PPARα) were purchased from Santa Cruz Biotechnology, Santa Cruz, CA, USA.

2.2. Cell Culture

Human hepatoma HepG2 cells were purchased from the American Type Culture Collection (ATCC, Manassas, VA, USA). The cells were grown at 37 °C, 5% CO_2, and 95% humidity in Dulbecco's modified Eagle's medium containing 50% [$U^{13}C6$]-glucose and

50% unlabeled glucose (100 mg/dL or 5.5 mM final concentration). HepG2 cells were serum-starved for 12 h, then were left untreated (HepG2 control) or exposed to oleic acid (OA, 0.5 μM) conjugated to bovine serum albumin (2:1) to induce steatosis. OA-exposed cells were treated with DMSO (OA-steatotic control), morin (10 μM), naringenin (10 μM), silibinin (10 μM), or topiramate (44 μM) for 72 h. The flavonoid concentrations were selected based on a literature review and were tested in our laboratory to confirm glucose utilization. A pharmacokinetic study in humans after ingestion of 135 mg oral naringenin resulted in a blood levels ranging from 7–9 μM [21]. The silibinin dose was chosen due to low or undetectable reported levels in human clinical trials and to avoid the apoptosis and reduction of glucose consumption seen in hepatocyte cell culture at a higher doses up to 200 μM [22]. Morin treatment has been published at dose ranges of 10–25 μM in hepatocyte cell cultures [9,10]. The topiramate concentration was selected based on published data using 44 uM as an approximation of physiologic concentrations ex vivo [23]. After the experimental period, cells were harvested, medium was collected, and samples were stored at −80 degree Celsius until being extracted for analysis. Figure 1 illustrates the timeline of the cell culture.

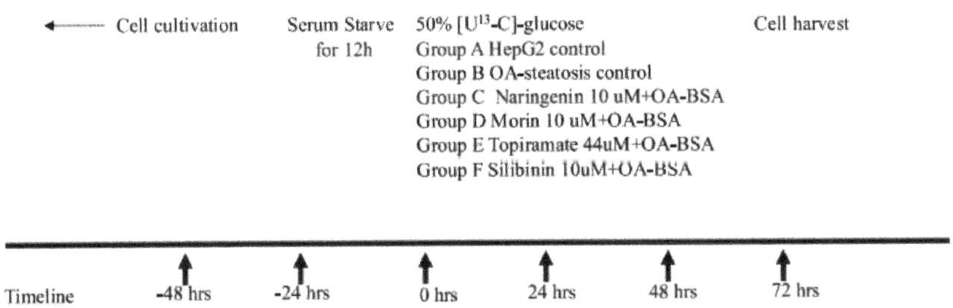

Figure 1. Timeline of cell culture experiment. After seeding and growing HepG2 cells in flasks, cells were serum-starved for 12 h, then were left untreated (HepG2 control) or were exposed to oleic acid (OA, 0.5 μM) conjugated to bovine serum albumin (2:1) to induce steatosis for 72 h. OA-exposed cells were also treated with one of the following compounds: DMSO (OA-exposed steatotic control), morin (10 μM), naringenin (10 μM), silibinin (10 μM), or topiramate (44 μM) for 72 h. Cell culture medium included 50% uniformly labeled glucose ($U^{13}C$-glucose) as a stable isotope tracer and was replaced every 24 h for the duration of the experiment. At 72 h, the cells were harvested as pellets for extraction and analysis of metabolites.

2.3. *Lipid Droplet Staining*

Lipid droplet staining was performed to quantify lipid accumulation in the cell culture model. An Oil Red O Staining Kit was used according to the manufacturer's protocol. Cells were grown in a 24-well plate, and treated as above for 48 h. The stained cells were incubated in 250 mL 60% isopropanol and absorbance was measured at 490 nm.

2.4. *Glucose Depletion from Cell Culture Medium*

HepG2 cells were grown in high-glucose medium in 96-well plates according to the treatment groups as above. Medium was collected at 24, 48, and 72 h, and glucose concentrations were determined using glucose oxidase/peroxidase reagent (Enzymatic Assay Kits). The sensitivity of this assay was sufficient for the expected concentrations in the medium. One mL glucose oxidase/peroxidase reagent was added to ten μL cell culture medium from each sample, then incubated at 37 °C for 10 min. HPLC-grade water was used as a blank, and the control standard was glucose 5.55 mM. The plates were read at 505 nm

(Molecular Devices). Glucose depletion from medium was determined by subtracting the glucose concentration from samples from the original medium concentration.

$$\text{Glucose (mM)} = (\text{Au Group-Au Blank})/(\text{Au Standard-Au Blank}) \times \text{Standard mM}.$$

2.5. Glycogen Production

Glucose is phosphorylated to glucose-6-phosphate which can be used toward glycogen synthesis for storage in hepatocytes. Glycogenosis has been observed in human MASLD [24]. Cell pellets were sonicated and extracted for analysis using previously published methods [25]. The isotopomer mass ratio of m/z 328 for the glucose derivative fragment was monitored and the SIGmn was calculated to represent the enrichment of glycogen from labeled glucose.

2.6. Fatty Acid Analysis: De Novo Synthesis, Desaturation, and Elongation

Aside from glycogen production, glucose-6-phosphate enters glycolysis to produce pyruvate, which is used as a substrate to enter the TCA cycle toward fatty acid synthesis. The GC/MS platform was used to analyze total (labeled + unlabeled) fatty acid composition, as well as incorporation of ^{13}C to determine the newly synthesized fraction of fatty acids.

Cell pellets were saponified to extract fatty acids from all lipid molecular species including triglycerides, cholesterol esters, and phospholipids. Cell pellets were treated in 30% KOH (w/v) and 100% ethanol overnight at 70 degrees Celsius. Fatty acids were extracted using petroleum ether, dried under nitrogen, then were derivatized as methyl esters using 0.5 N methanolic-HCl. Analysis was performed on an Agilent 6890 N gas chromatograph coupled with a model 5975 mass spectrometer detector system. For this, 1 µL samples were injected by the automatic sampler, with each biological replicate run in duplicate or triplicate for precision. The GC column used was a Bpx70 column (30 m length × 250 µm diameter × 0.25 µm film thickness) (SGE, Inc., Austin, TX, USA). GC conditions were as follows: helium flow rate, 1 mL/min; oven temperature was initially set at 150 °C, and programmed to increase at 3 °C/min to a final temperature of 221 °C. Using known standards for comparison, palmitate was identified at a retention time of 5.1 min, palmitoleic at 5.5 min, stearate at 7.4 min, oleate at 7.9 min, vaccenate at 8.0 min, and linoleic at 8.8 min. Mass spectra were acquired using electron impact ionization and selective ion monitoring at m/z 270 for palmitate, m/z of 298 for stearate, and m/z 296 for oleate. Acetyl-CoA enrichment and de novo lipogenesis were determined from the mass isotopomer distribution of palmitate, stearate, and oleate as reported previously [26]. Peak integrations were performed on the background subtracted spectra from total ion chromatogram using Chemstation software (Agilent, Palo Alto, CA, USA).

Fatty acids produced by de novo synthesis may undergo further modifications. The relative rates of conversion over the experiment were estimated by calculating their precursor-to-product ratios [27,28]. Delta-9 desaturation of stearate to oleate is represented by the oleate/stearate desaturation index, calculated by dividing the fraction of new oleate synthesis by the fraction of new palmitate synthesis. Elongation of palmitate to stearate was calculated by dividing the fraction of new stearate synthesis by the fraction of new palmitate synthesis.

2.7. Glutamate

Pyruvate undergoes carboxylation into oxaloacetate for entry into the tricarboxylic acid (TCA) cycle via pyruvate carboxylase (PC) or undergoes decarboxylation via the pyruvate dehydrogenase (PDH) pathway to produce acetyl-CoA. Glutamate can be studied by isotopomer analysis for PC vs. PDH pathway contributions because it equilibrates with α-ketoglutarate, a key intermediate in the TCA cycle. ^{13}C is incorporated in a signature pattern based on PC vs. PDH entry. Cell pellets underwent sonication, and extracts were precipitated in 30% ethanol. The supernatant fractions containing the amino acids were dried under a nitrogen stream. Glutamate was derivatized using n-trifluoroacetyl-n-butyl ester (TAB). GC/MS analysis was performed using a 6890 gas chromatograph and Hewlett-Packard 5973 N mass spectrometer with electron impact ionization. The GC column used was a 30 m ZB5® (Phenomenex) capillary column [29]. The GC program was as follows: injector temperature 250 °C; oven temperature started at 170 °C for 2 min initially, then rose by 3 °C/min to 190 °C and 40 °C/min to an ultimate temperature of 270 °C. Helium supplied the carrier gas at 1 mL/min. The retention time of glutamate was 11.69 min. Selected ion monitoring (SIM) identified two fragments, m/z 198 and 152, corresponding to the C2–C5 and C2–C4 fragments of glutamate [30]. The isotopomer distribution was used, as previously published, to determine the pathways from which glutamate was produced [29].

Glutamate with labeled carbon at positions 4–5 results from pyruvate dehydrogenase (PDH) pathway activity, while glutamate with labeled carbon on the 2–3 positions reflects pyruvate carboxylase (PC) activity when carbon enters the TCA cycle. When both carbons are labeled on the C2–C4 fragment (m^2 of m/z 152), this means the ^{13}C was incorporated through PC, while the m^2 isotopomer of the C2–C5 fragment (m/z 198) is evidence of ^{13}C entry via PC and PDH. The pyruvate carboxylase/pyruvate dehydrogenase (PC/PDH) ratio was previously published as (m^2 of m/z 152 fragment)/[(m^2 of m/z 198 fragment)-(m^2 of m/z 152 fragment)] to represent variation in pyruvate entry into the TCA cycle in the process of producing acetyl-CoA [29].

2.8. Cell Proliferation

Cell proliferation was determined using Cell Counting Kit-8 at 24, 48, and 72 h to determine cell survival of the treatments over the time course of the experiment. The proliferation data are complementary to the ribose synthesis data in screening for perturbations in cell replication or viability. The cells were seeded (3×10^3 cells) in a 96-well plate and treated as above. Cell proliferation was detected with CCK8 reagent. Ten μL Cell Counting Kit-8 reagent was added to each well, incubated with cells at 37 °C, 5% CO_2, and 95% humidity for 1 h, then plates were read at 450 nm with spectrophotometry (Molecular Devices SpectraMax Plus 384). Cell proliferation was calculated as a percent of the control group.

$$\text{Cell proliferation (\%)} = \text{A Group}/\text{A Control} \times 100.$$

2.9. RNA Ribose

Glucose-6-phosphate enters the pentose phosphate pathway to synthesize ribose for nucleotide production to support cellular replication. Ribose enrichment was analyzed as a reflection of cell proliferation. Trizol was used to treat cell pellets, then RNA ribose was extracted through acid hydrolysis of the chloroform-isopropanol layer. Ribose was derivatized using aldonitrile acetate, then analyzed with an HP 6890 gas chromatograph and 5973 mass spectrometer. Fragment m/z 256 (carbons 1–5 of ribose) was analyzed by mass isotopomer distribution analysis [31].

2.10. Western Blotting

Western blotting for SREBP1 and FAS was performed to assess for changes in lipogenic protein expression. PPARα protein expression was also investigated for potential changes in regulation of fatty oxidation. Cell pellets were sonicated in RIPA buffer with phosphodiesterase inhibitor and EDTA. Protein concentration was measured using the BCA Protein Assay (Pierce). Gel electrophoresis was performed using a precast BisTris gel (BioRad), then protein was transferred to nitrocellulose membranes. The membrane was treated with non-fat milk to block non-specific binding. Primary antibodies were applied overnight, membranes washed, and secondary antibodies applied. Bands were visualized by chemiluminescence (Pierce Super Signal West Pico Chemiluminescence kit) in a darkroom. Protein loading bands were identified by staining with Ponceau S. Densitometry was performed on the protein of interest and band intensities were normalized to the protein loading bands.

2.11. Statistical Analysis

SYSTAT software was used for statistical analysis. Groups were compared by ANOVA with post hoc pairwise comparisons using Tukey's test since sample sizes in groups were similar. The Shapiro–Wilk's test was used to confirm normal distribution of data. $p < 0.05$ was considered to indicate significant differences between treated groups compared to HepG2 control or OA-steatosis cells (steatosis control).

3. Results

3.1. Lipid Accumulation

Lipid accumulation was studied to confirm the efficacy of OA in inducing steatosis and the relative impact of flavonoid or topiramate as interventions. Untreated cells and OA-steatotic cells with DMSO or naringenin, morin, topiramate, or silibinin were studied for lipid accumulation by ORO staining after 48 h. Overall, the groups demonstrated significant differences ($p < 0.000001$). OA-steatotic cells with DMSO showed a 1.6-fold greater intensity of staining compared to untreated controls ($p < 0.001$). Compared to the OA-steatotic cells with DMSO, treatment with naringenin or morin showed similar absorbance, whereas topiramate treatment ($p = 0.0005$) or silibinin ($p = 0.0003$) demonstrated significantly lower absorbance (1.3-fold compared to untreated non-steatotic control). (Figure 2).

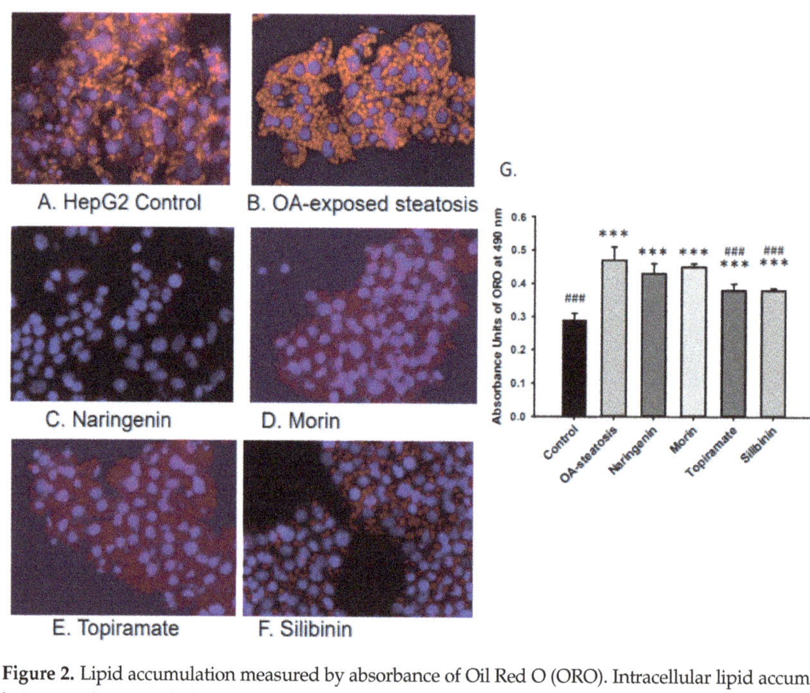

Figure 2. Lipid accumulation measured by absorbance of Oil Red O (ORO). Intracellular lipid accumulation was determined after ORO staining using a microplate reader. Data represents means ± standard deviation of the mean (SD) with $n = 6$ wells of cells for each group. Photos were taken at 40× magnification. (**A**). HepG2 untreated control, (**B**). OA-steatosis DMSO control, (**C**). naringenin-treated

steatotic cells, (**D**). morin-treated steatotic cells, (**E**). topiramate-treated steatotic cells, and (**F**). silibinin-treated steatotic cells. (**G**). Measured absorbance units (AU) of treatment groups stained with ORO measured at 490 nm. Compared to HepG2 controls: *** $p < 0.001$. Compared to the OA-steatosis group: ### $p < 0.001$.

3.2. Glucose Depletion from Cell Culture Medium

Glucose depletion was determined from medium (replaced daily) at 24, 48, and 72 h to assess for overall glucose utilization. Glucose depletion increased daily. No differences were observed among treatment groups at 24 h (aggregate mean 7.2 ± 1.8 mmol/L), or 72 h (aggregate mean 12.6 ± 2.2 mmol/L). At 48 h, differences among the groups were observed: untreated cells 11.4 ± 1.5 mmol/L, OA-exposed steatosis group 12.1 ± 1.0 mmol/L, naringenin-treated 11.5.0 ± 2.6 mmol/L, morin-treated 14.0 ± 1.7 mmol/L, topiramate-treated 11.8 ± 3.6 mmol/L, silibinin-treated 7.1 ± 3.2, $p < 0.0015$). In pair-wise testing, glucose depletion in the silibinin-treated group was significantly lower than in the OA-exposed steatotic group.

3.3. Glycogen Production

Glycogen synthesis is one of the three major pathway destinations for glucose-6-phosphate. Glycogenosis has been observed in MASLD in humans [24] as a sign of metabolic dysfunction, and this study examined ^{13}C enrichment to detect changes in glycogen production. The isotopomer mass ratio of m/z 328 for the glucose derivative fragment was monitored and the SIGmn was calculated to represent the enrichment of glycogen from labeled glucose. At 72 h, the SIGmn was 1.65 ± 0.06 for controls, 1.55 ± 0.07 in OA-exposed steatotic cells, 1.41 ± 0.03 in steatotic cells treated with morin, 1.55 ± 0.07 in steatotic cells treated with naringenin, 1.68 ± 0.08 in steatosis cells treated with topiramate, and 1.40 ± 0.10 in steatosis cells treated with silibinin. No significant difference was identified among the groups ($p = 0.053$).

3.4. Fatty Acid Analysis

3.4.1. Long Chain Fatty Acid Profile

Fatty acids stored in liver triglycerides are largely comprised of long chain fatty acids. The total fatty acid composition includes preexisting fatty acids, those taken up from exogenous sources, and those from de novo synthesis. Cell groups were first analyzed for total long chain fatty acid composition, including labeled and unlabeled species. Figure 3A shows the major long chain fatty acids, palmitate (16:0), palmitoleate (16:1n-7), stearate (18:0), oleate (18:1n-9), and vaccenate (18:1n-7), from our samples. Linoleate, which is an essential n-6 fatty acid, had very low abundance, 1.81 ± 0.06% in HelpG2 controls and <1% in most, but not all, of the samples in the steatosis groups. n-3 fatty acids were in even lower abundance. Analysis by ANOVA showed significant differences among all groups for each of these fatty acids ($p < 0.001$). Compared to baseline control cells, OA-steatosis demonstrated decreased abundance in palmitate, palmitoleate, stearate, and vaccenate. There was an increase in abundance of oleate, which is likely due to uptake from the exogenous supply. Topiramate and silibinin both maintained the pattern seen in OA-steatosis. Compared to the OA-steatosis group, morin-treated cells had higher abundance of palmitate and lower oleate, while naringenin-treated cells had higher abundance of palmitoleate and lower oleate.

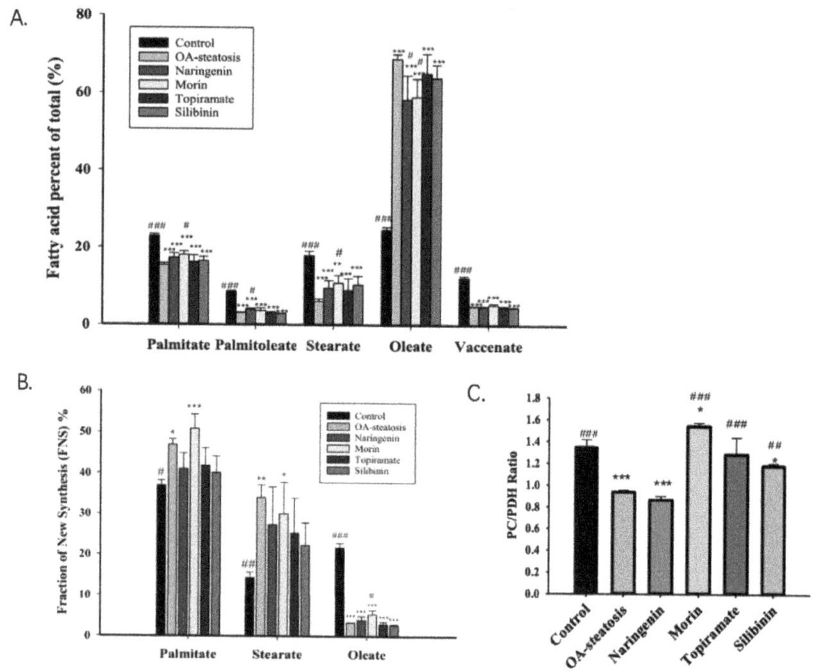

Figure 3. The fatty acid profile, palmitate de novo synthesis, and the pyruvate carboxylase/pyruvate dehydrogenase ratio. Fatty acids stored in liver are largely comprised of long chain fatty acids. (**A**). The abundance of the major long chain fatty acids (labeled + unlabeled) is presented as the percent of total (%) with mean and standard deviation (SD). The OA-steatotic groups exhibited oleate in the highest abundance. (**B**). The Fraction of New Synthesis (FNS), expressed as a percent, represents the de novo fatty acid synthesis rate over the 72 h experiment and is calculated from the incorporation of ^{13}C. The FNS is shown for palmitate, stearate, and oleate. OA-steatotic cells demonstrated higher FNS palmitate and stearate. This difference was ameliorated by naringenin, topiramate, and silibinin. With or without treatment, OA-steatosis resulted in suppressed FNS oleate. Morin mildly raised the FNS oleate. (**C**). The pyruvate carboxylase/pyruvate dehydrogenase (PC/PDH) ratio in arbitrary units represents the relative contribution of the two pathways to de novo synthesis. Compared to HepG2 controls: * $p < 0.05$, ** $p < 0.01$, *** $p < 0.001$. Compared to the OA-steatosis group: # $p < 0.05$, ## $p < 0.01$, ### $p < 0.001$.

3.4.2. De Novo Synthesis of Fatty Acids

Glucose-6-phosphate enters glycolysis to produce pyruvate that enters the TCA cycle to contribute toward de novo fatty acid synthesis. Palmitate (16:0) is the main product of de novo synthesis, produced from acetyl-CoA and malonyl-CoA by acetyl-CoA carboxylase and fatty acid synthase (FAS). Stearate (18:0) may be produced de novo or from chain elongation of preexisting palmitate, and oleate is produced by desaturation of stearate. The measurement of newly made fatty acids incorporating the ^{13}C isotope over time is the fraction of new synthesis (FNS) expressed as a percent. ANOVA analysis determined an overall difference among the groups for palmitate ($p = 0.00087$), stearate ($p = 0.01$), and oleate ($p < 0.001$). In comparison to untreated control cells, OA-exposed steatotic cells showed an increased palmitate FNS rate ($p = 0.002$), which persisted with morin treatment. Notably, this significant increase was ameliorated in groups treated with naringenin, topiramate, and silibinin, with the FNS rates showing variation and overlap with the untreated control as well (Figure 3B). For FNS stearate, a similar pattern was shown among groups; however, a high degree of variation suggested additional factors affecting the newly synthesized stearate pool. For FNS oleate, the OA-steatosis and treatments groups all demonstrated lower rates than the untreated control. Notably, morin treatment resulted in slightly higher rates than in OA-steatosis. Acetyl-CoA enrichment was similar in all groups (baseline control 0.19 ± 0.01, OA-exposed steatosis 0.19 ± 0.00, steatotic cells treated with naringenin 0.19 ± 0.01, morin 0.19 ± 00, topiramate 0.19 ± 0.01, or silibinin 0.20 ± 0.01).

3.4.3. The Desaturation Index and Elongation Index

Liver triglycerides often include at least one unsaturated fatty acid, such as oleate. Oleate is produced by delta-9 desaturation of stearate, while stearate is produced by de novo synthesis or elongation from palmitate. These processes, which impact metabolite pool size, can be reflected in the calculation of the precursor-to-product ratios. The new oleate/stearate ratio and the new stearate/palmitate ratio represent the desaturation index and elongation index, respectively (Table 1). The desaturation index was significantly different among groups ($p << 0.001$), with all steatosis groups exhibiting similarly low indices compared to the HepG2 control. The elongation index also differed among groups ($p = 0.01$). OA-steatotic cells had higher elongation indices, while naringenin maintained the higher rates. Morin, topiramate, and silibinin treatments result in variable indices that overlapped both the HepG2 control and OA-steatosis groups. Taken together, OA-induced steatosis results in suppression of delta-9 desaturation, leading to accumulation of de novo synthesized fatty acids.

Table 1. Desaturation and elongation. The ratio of new oleate/stearate represents delta 9 desaturation of stearate to produce monounsaturated oleate. The ratio of new stearate/palmitate reflects chain elongation of 16-carbon palmitate to 18-carbon stearate. Ratios are shown as mean values with the standard deviation. Compared to HepG2 controls: * $p < 0.05$, ** $p < 0.01$, *** $p < 0.001$. Compared to the OA-steatosis group: ## $p < 0.01$, ### $p < 0.001$.

Fatty Acid Ratio	Control	OA-Steatosis	Naringenin	Morin	Topiramate	Silibinin
Oleate/stearate desaturation index	1.53 ± 0.14 ###	0.10 ± 0.01 ***	0.17 ± 0.09 ***	0.19 ± 0.07 ***	0.13 ± 0.07 ***	0.13 ± 0.03 ***
Stearate/palmitate elongation index	0.39 ± 0.02 ##	0.72 ± 0.05 **	0.65 ± 0.16 *	0.59 ± 0.10	0.59 ± 0.16	0.55 ± 0.09

3.4.4. Western Blotting of SREBP1, FAS, and PPARα

SREBP is a transcription factor that induces lipogenic gene expression. The enzyme FAS catalyzes fatty acid synthesis from acetyl coA and malonyl coA. Transcription factor PPARα promotes expression of genes involved in fatty acid oxidation. Western blotting was performed to determine whether protein expression of the above regulators contributed to the findings in this cell culture model. No changes in protein expression of SREBP1, FAS, or PPARα were observed (Figure 4). This leaves open the possibility of post-translational effects such as enzyme activity that contributed to the differences in de novo synthesis.

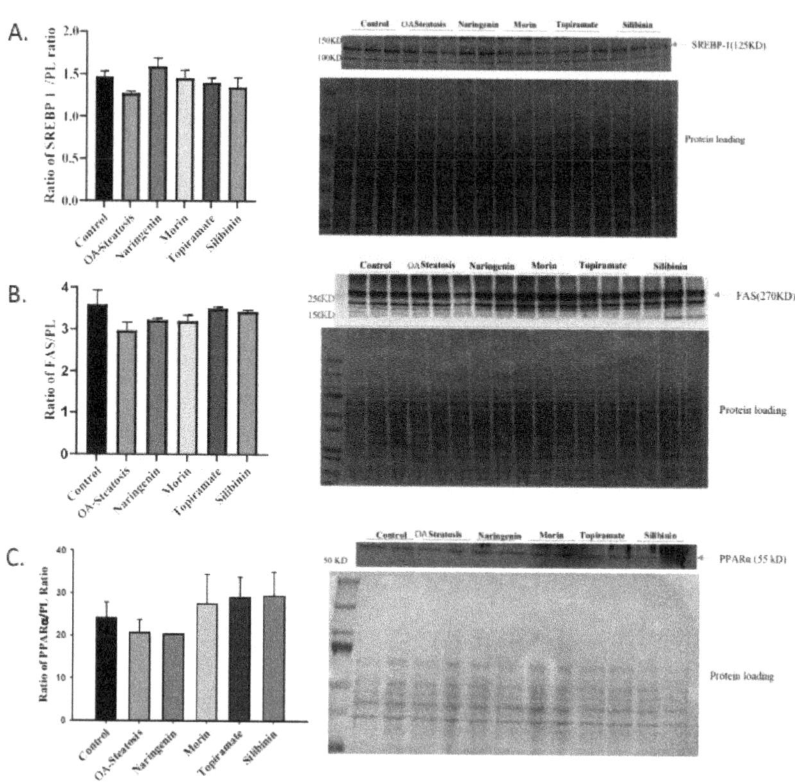

Figure 4. Western blotting of SREBP, FAS, and PPARα. Western blotting was performed on protein extracted from cell pellets. Signal intensity was analyzed relative to that of protein loading bands.

3.5. The Pyruvate Carboxylase/Pyruvate Dehydrogenase Ratio and TCA Cycle Activity

Pyruvate enters the mitochondria and contributes to the TCA cycle through two pathways. The pyruvate carboxylase pathway produces OAA, promotes gluconeogenesis, and counteracts oxidative stress through glutathione and NADPH synthesis. Pyruvate dehydrogenase produces acetyl-CoA for de novo synthesis. Glutamate enrichment in the 4–5 carbon positions was analyzed for pyruvate dehydrogenase (PDH) activity, while glutamate enriched on the 2–3 carbon positions was analyzed for pyruvate carboxylase (PC) activity for entry into the TCA cycle. The PC/PDH ratio is a reflection of the relative contribution of each pathway to the TCA cycle. Compared to untreated control cells (1.35 ± 0.07), OA-induced steatosis reduced the ratio, (0.94 ± 0.02, $p < 0.001$). In comparison to the OA-steatosis group, the ratio was maintained by naringenin treatment (0.87 ± 0.03). whereas morin (1.55 ± 0.03, $p < 0.001$), topiramate (1.29 ± 0.16, $p < 0.001$), and silibinin (1.18 ± 0.02, $p = 0.002$) promoted higher ratios (Figure 3C).

3.6. Cell Proliferation

The groups of cells showed no differences among them and exhibited full proliferation at each time point. At 72 h, values were control 100.0 ± 1.2%, OA-steatosis 100.0 ± 1.3%, naringenin 100 ± 3.9%, morin 100 ± 2.9%, topiramate 100 ± 9.9%, and silibinin 100 ± 2.3%.

3.7. RNA-Ribose Synthesis

One of the three major pathways of entry by glucose-6-phosphate is the pentose phosphate pathway (PPP). The PPP produces nucleotides necessary for cell replication activities. The incorporation of ^{13}C from glucose reflects RNA-ribose new synthesis activities. The contribution of glucose carbon to ribose is calculated by determining the ^{13}C molar enrichment in ribose (Figure 5). OA treatment (1.46 ± 0.001) significantly lowered ribose synthesis when compared to the untreated control (1.54 ± 0.001, $p = 0.002$). Compared to the OA-steatotic cells, silibinin (1.41 ± 0.001) and topiramate (1.43 ± 0.001) did not change the rate, while morin further lowered it (1.29 ± 0.03, $p < 0.001$). Naringenin (1.49 ± 0.03) enrichment was not different from either control cells or the OA-steatosis cells.

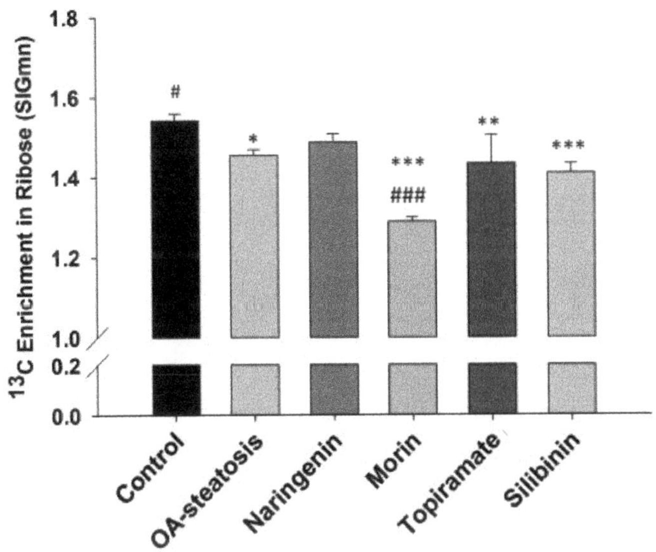

Figure 5. ^{13}C Enrichment in ribose (SIGmn). Glucose-6-phosphate enters the pentose phosphate pathway (PPP) for production of nucleotides to support cell replication. Ribose production reflects PPP activity. The ^{13}C molar enrichment in ribose represents ribose synthesis over the time course of the experiment. In OA-steatosis, ribose synthesis is lower than when compared to the non-steatotic untreated control ($p = 0.002$). Compared to HepG2 controls: * $p < 0.05$, ** $p < 0.01$, *** $p < 0.001$. Compared to the OA-steatosis group: # $p < 0.05$, ### $p < 0.001$.

3.8. Results Summary

An OA-induced steatosis cell culture model was created in HepG2 cells to study the contribution of glucose to carbon metabolic pathways and impact of flavonoids or topiramate as interventions. The steatotic cells demonstrated lipid accumulation by ORO and robust cell proliferation. Using U^{13}C-glucose, relative pathway analysis of outcomes from the three major destinations for glucose-6-phosphate were studied, showing that OA-steatosis was associated with lower ribose synthesis from the PPP, no change in glycogen synthesis, enhanced new synthesis of palmitate and stearate, increased elongation, and lower desaturation to oleate. (Figure 6, Table 2). Interventions showed some mitigation of lipid accumulation by topiramate and silibinin and mitigation in enhancement of de novo synthesis and the PC/PDH ratio. Naringenin treatment resulted in persistently enhanced elongation and improved ribose synthesis. Morin-treated cells showed enhanced de novo synthesis of saturated fatty acids, as well as oleate.

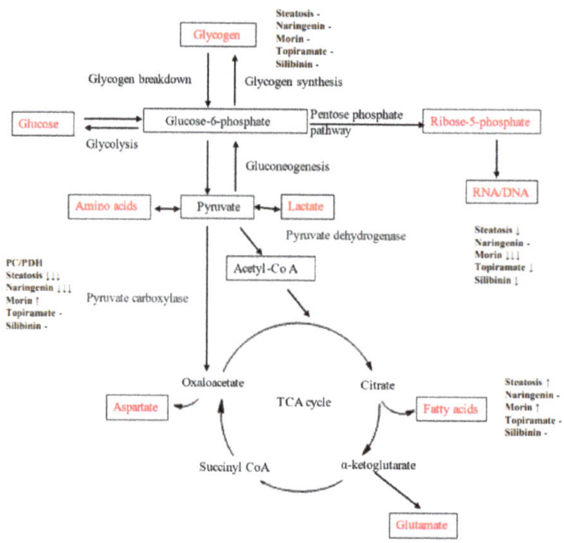

Figure 6. Diagram of metabolic pathways through which carbon flux occurs. Direction of change in OA-steatotic cells and their treatment groups is indicated at each measured metabolic outcome, relative to non-steatotic, untreated HepG2 cells.

Table 2. Summary of changes noted in metabolic pathways studied. The untreated HepG2 group is the reference control group.

Metabolic Pathway	Control	OA-Steatosis	Naringenin	Morin	Topiramate	Silibinin
Glycogen	reference	-	-	-	-	-
Palmitate and stearate de novo synthesis	reference	increased	-	increased	-	-
Delta-9 desaturation	reference	decreased	decreased	decreased	decreased	decreased
Elongation	reference	increased	increased	-	-	-
PC/PDH ratio	reference	greatly decreased	greatly decreased	increased	-	-
Ribose synthesis	reference	decreased	-	greatly decreased	decreased	decreased

4. Discussion

This study was designed to investigate the effects of three flavonoids and topiramate on glucose-derived carbon flux in a HepG2 cell culture model of steatosis. We examined outcomes related to three main pathways through which glucose enters as glucose-6-phosphate: glycogen synthesis, the pentose phosphate pathway, and glycolysis, which produces pyruvate to enter the mitochondria into the TCA cycle. For the interventions, unlike many in vitro studies that have used high doses, we used relatively low doses (flavonoids 10 μM, topiramate 44 μM) that are physiologically relevant to the concentrations found in human blood after ingestion. For example, serum concentrations of naringenin in healthy subjects who ingested a single dose of 150 mg naringenin were found to be 15.76 ± 7.88 μM [21].

Oleic and palmitic acid are the most abundant fatty acids in hepatic triglycerides. Change in fatty acid composition through de novo synthesis or turnover may contribute to the pathogenesis of MASLD [32]. Oleic acid has been shown to be more steatotic than palmitic acid [33] and to promote reactive oxygen species (ROS) production and TNFα expression [34], which contribute to the progression of MASLD to MASH. OA-exposed HepG2 hepatocytes were often employed as an in vitro model of steatosis to investigate the molecular mechanisms underlying MASLD [34,35]. Results from our study indicated that OA-exposed cells significantly increased intracellular lipid accumulation, consistent with published data [35], and demonstrated ample cell proliferation. Relative pathway analyses in OA-steatotic cells showed no effect on glycogen synthesis, with lower ribose synthesis rate but higher de novo synthesis. Together with higher elongation and suppressed desaturation, the fatty acid pathways are shifted toward synthesis and accumulation of new saturated fatty acids, promoting a lipid composition for storage. A similar shift was previously reported in an alcohol-induced rat model of liver disease [28], supporting triglyceride storage and reduced export. The lower PC/PDH ratio suggests a relative increase in PDH activity.

The observation of the lower PC/PDH ratio in our OA-steatotic cells contrasts with previously published studies on the PC and PDH activities in MASLD. Mice with high-fat-diet-induced hepatic steatosis demonstrated benefits from having enhanced PDH activity from inhibition of pyruvate dehydrogenase kinase 2 and decreased PC flux through increased fatty acid oxidation and ketone body formation [36]. A tracer study on TCA cycle activity in humans with MASLD supported higher activity through PC [37]. Therefore, we speculate that our finding of lower PC/PDH might reflect a metabolic adaptive response under our artificial cell culture system rather than intrinsic dysfunction in rodent models and in human disease.

In our study, we found that silibinin exposure significantly reduced lipid accumulation in OA-steatotic HepG2 cells. Silibinin-treated cells did not demonstrate the increase in de novo synthesis rate that was observed in untreated OA-steatotic cells. These results suggest that silibinin could potentially ameliorate lipid accumulation induced by OA in HepG2 cells. The increase in PC/PDH ratio with sibilinin treatment suggests a restoration of the balance between the two pathways. Although SREBP1, FAS, and PPARα protein expression appeared unchanged in all groups including silibinin, the protein expression is a static marker of activity at the end of the experiment, whereas the FNS represents the accumulation of de novo synthesis over the course of 72 h. Silibinin treatment maintained the diminished ribose synthesis seen in OA-steatotic cells, which suggests an inability to correct nucleotide imbalance. A reciprocal relationship between the inhibition of the de novo lipogenesis (palmitate synthesis) and the inhibition of ribose/deoxyribose has been noted in several studies [17,31,38].

Silibinin is the only compound investigated that demonstrated decreased glucose depletion from the medium, but only at the 48 h time point. The dose of silibinin used in this experiment was relatively low compared to published data showing that silibinin treatment (20–100 μM) increases glucose uptake and decreases intracellular triglyceride in OA-treated HepG2 cells [39]. The published study also demonstrates that silibinin can ameliorate some metabolic alterations and induce some molecular changes by activating the Caspase 8 and Fas-associated protein with death domain-like apoptosis regulator and c-Jun N-terminal kinase (CFLAR-JNK) pathway, thereby regulating its downstream target genes involved in lipid metabolism (PPARα, SREBP-1c, and PNPLA3), glucose uptake (PI3K-AKT), oxidative stress (NRF2, CYP2E1, and CYP4A), and inflammatory response (NO) in OA-treated HepG2 cells. Most of these effects were observed at doses of 50 μM or higher [35], so dose-dependent variation is possible. The overall profile of silibinin has also been described as a mimetic for the fasting state through promotion of the AMPK pathway and inhibition of glycolysis [22].

Treatment with other flavonoids impacted metabolic pathways differently, and with less success in lipid accumulation. Although a published study by Gu et al. found that morin mitigated triglyceride (TG) accumulation in OA-induced HepG2 cells [9], morin did not overtly affect lipid accumulation in our study, possibly due to the relatively low dose used. On the other hand, in comparison to the OA-steatosis group, morin treatment notably maintained similarly high FNS palmitate and stearate rates, but this was also the only intervention group to demonstrate a higher FNS oleate. Despite appearing very lipogenic, the restoration of PC/PDH to be similar to HepG2 controls suggests some improvement of phenotype mediated by morin. A benefit of the PC pathway includes protection from oxidative stress through glutathione synthesis, which removes ROS that may cause inflammation and cell damage. A published hepatocyte cell culture study on glucotoxicity-induced liver damage showed that morin was protective through reduction of ROS [40]. Whether morin's antioxidant effects are attributable to PC activity in MASLD requires future research. On the other hand, naringenin promoted ribose synthesis, but maintained a lower PC/PDH ratio similar to the OA-steatosis group. It is possible that naringenin is protective against hepatocyte steatosis via enhancing ribose synthesis to support nucleotide balance. Naringenin may have potential benefits in pathways not studied here. In mice with MASLD induced by methionine-choline deficiency and in HpeG2 cells treated with OA, naringenin reduced lipid accumulation through inhibition of the inflammatory cytokine-mediated signaling pathway NLRP3/NFkB [41].

Topiramate is a potent antiepileptic drug whose side effects of weight loss in patients with epilepsy and obesity led to the FDA approval of this drug combined with phentermine as an anti-obesity medication. Topiramate has been studied more for its insulin sensitizing and weight control properties, and less is known about its effects on MASLD. A study of the effects of topiramate in female Zucker diabetic fatty (ZDF) rats demonstrated that topiramate treatment leads to a decrease in hepatic glucose output, increased insulin sensitivity in adipose but not muscle, and suppression of adipose tissue lipolysis [23]. The study focused largely on actions in adipocytes and muscle. Although MASLD was not studied explicitly, topiramate treatment in rats with high-fat/high-fructose-induced insulin resistance resulted in increased liver expression of adiponectin receptors, GLUT2, and tyrosine kinase activity [16], thereby implicating pathways of glucose utilization and cell proliferation. Our study contributes toward filling the knowledge gap regarding topiramate's effects on MASLD, showing that topiramate may counteract OA-steatosis by inhibiting lipid accumulation, in association with some abatement of enhanced de novo synthesis and improvement in the PC/PDH balance.

Limitations of this study include the use of single doses of each compound, so information was not obtained on dose-dependent effects. Use of $U^{13}C$-glucose as the tracer did not permit separate examination of the transketolase and transaldolase pathways in the ribose analysis. Western blotting determined protein expression only, which leaves open the possibility of post-translational effects. This study focused on carbon metabolism derived from glucose and does not address all systems affected by steatosis (e.g., ER stress and inflammation) or potential interplay between organ systems. Cell culture systems such as this OA-induced model do not completely replicate the physiology of MASLD seen in human subjects.

5. Conclusions

In this OA-induced HepG2 cell culture model of liver steatosis, glucose utilization was associated with decreased ribose synthesis, enhanced de novo synthesis, and suppression of desaturation to oleate, all reflecting relative pathway activities favoring lipid storage. A ^{13}C tracer analysis allowed the detection of small but significant differences in pathway activities among cells treated with flavonoids or topiramate. Silibinin and topiramate decreased lipid accumulation and mitigated enhancement of de novo synthesis. Morin treatment appeared to favor de novo synthesis pathways, drawing glucose-derived carbons aways from ribose synthesis. Since the doses used were based on levels relevant to human exposure, the mild effects observed in our study could be consistent with the variation of effects in human disease. Future preclinical or clinical studies could explore how short-term vs. long-term treatment affects these pathways. Additional studies would be useful to investigate whether the treatment is effective at various stages of MASLD, including for MASLD prevention and the more advanced stages leading up to MASH.

Author Contributions: Conceptualization, L.M., Q.-Y.L., L.G.B. and J.K.Y.; methodology, L.M. and S.L.; software, L.G.B. and J.K.Y.; validation, L.M. and J.K.Y.; formal analysis, L.M. and J.K.Y.; investigation, L.M., S.L. and G.H.; resources, L.M., M.D. and J.K.Y.; data curation, L.M. and J.K.Y.; writing—original draft preparation, L.M., Q.-Y.L. and J.K.Y.; Writing—review, editing, approval, L.M., Q.-Y.L., L.G.B., J.K.Y., M.D., S.L. and G.H.; visualization, L.M.; supervision, M.D. and J.K.Y.; project administration, J.K.Y.; funding acquisition, L.M. and J.K.Y. All authors have read and agreed to the published version of the manuscript.

Funding: This project was supported in part by a Core Voucher from The Lundquist Institute of Biomedical Innovation at Harbor-UCLA Medical Center, funded through the University of California Los Angeles Clinical and Translational Science Institute, NIH NCATS grant number UL1TR001881.

Institutional Review Board Statement: Not applicable.

Informed Consent Statement: Not applicable.

Data Availability Statement: The dataset is available on request from the authors.

Acknowledgments: This manuscript is dedicated to the memory of Wai-Nang Paul Lee.

Conflicts of Interest: The authors declare no conflicts of interest. The funding source had no role in the design of the study; in the collection, analyses, or interpretation of data; in the writing of the manuscript; or in the decision to publish the results.

Abbreviations

The following abbreviations are used in this manuscript:

OA	Oleic acid
MASLD	Metabolic dysfunction-associated steatotic liver disease
MASH	Metabolic-dysfunction-associated steatohepatitis
TCA	Tricarboxylic acid cycle
PC/PDH	Pyruvate carboxylase/pyruvate dehydrogenase

References

1. Mazhar, K. The Future of Nonalcoholic Fatty Liver Disease Treatment. *Med. Clin. N. Am.* **2019**, *103*, 57–69. [CrossRef] [PubMed]
2. Rinella, M.E. Nonalcoholic Fatty Liver Disease: A Systematic Review. *JAMA* **2015**, *313*, 2263–2273. [CrossRef] [PubMed]
3. Wang, R.; Yan, R.; Jiao, J.; Li, F.; Zhang, H.; Chang, Z.; Wei, H.; Yan, S.; Li, J. Fruit and vegetable intake and the risk of non-alcoholic fatty liver disease: A meta-analysis of observational studies. *Front. Nutr.* **2024**, *11*, 1398184. [CrossRef] [PubMed]
4. Kositamongkol, C.; Kanchanasurakit, S.; Auttamalang, C.; Inchai, N.; Kabkaew, T.; Kitpark, S.; Chaiyakunapruk, N.; Duangjai, A.; Saokaew, S.; Phisalprapa, P. Coffee Consumption and Non-Alcoholic Fatty Liver Disease: An Umbrella Review and a Systematic Review and Meta-Analysis. *Front. Pharmacol.* **2021**, *12*, 786596. [CrossRef]
5. Mansour-Ghanaei, F.; Hadi, A.; Pourmasoumi, M.; Joukar, F.; Golpour, S.; Najafgholizadeh, A. Green Tea as a Safe Alternative Approach for Nonalcoholic Fatty Liver Treatment: A Systematic Review and Meta-Analysis of Clinical Trials. *Phytother. Res.* **2018**, *32*, 1876–1884. [CrossRef]

6. Naeini, F.; Namkhah, Z.; Ostadrahimi, A.; Tutunchi, H.; Hosseinzadeh-Attar, M.J. A Comprehensive Systematic Review on the Effects of Naringenin, a Citrus-Derived Flavonoid, on Risk Factors for Nonalcoholic Fatty Liver Disease. *Adv. Nutr.* **2021**, *12*, 413–428. [CrossRef]
7. Federico, A.; Dallio, M.; Loguercio, C. Silymarin/Silybin and Chronic Liver Disease: A Marriage of Many Years. *Molecules* **2017**, *22*, 191. [CrossRef]
8. Loguercio, C.; Andreone, P.; Brisc, C.; Brisc, M.C.; Bugianesi, E.; Chiaramonte, M.; Cursaro, C.; Danila, M.; de Sio, I.; Floreani, A.; et al. Silybin Combined with Phosphatidylcholine and Vitamin E in Patients with Nonalcoholic Fatty Liver Disease: A Randomized Controlled Trial. *Free Radic. Biol. Med.* **2012**, *52*, 1658–1665. [CrossRef]
9. Gu, M.; Zhang, Y.; Liu, C.; Wang, D.; Feng, L.; Fan, S.; Yang, B.; Tong, Q.; Ji, G.; Huang, C. Morin, a Novel Liver X Receptor A/B Dual Antagonist, Has Potent Therapeutic Efficacy for Nonalcoholic Fatty Liver Diseases. *Br. J. Pharmacol.* **2017**, *174*, 3032–3044. [CrossRef]
10. Wu, L.; Wang, Y.; Chi, G.; Shen, B.; Tian, Y.; Li, Z.; Han, L.; Zhang, Q.; Feng, H. Morin Reduces Inflammatory Responses and Alleviates Lipid Accumulation in Hepatocytes. *J. Cell. Physiol.* **2019**, *234*, 19785–19798. [CrossRef]
11. Gillessen, A.; Schmidt, H.H. Silymarin as Supportive Treatment in Liver Diseases: A Narrative Review. *Adv. Ther.* **2020**, *37*, 1279–1301. [CrossRef] [PubMed]
12. Tan, P.; Jin, L.; Qin, X.; He, B. Natural Flavonoids: Potential Therapeutic Strategies for Non-Alcoholic Fatty Liver Disease. *Front. Pharmacol.* **2022**, *13*, 1005312. [CrossRef] [PubMed]
13. Wilding, J.; Van Gaal, L.; Rissanen, A.; Vercruysse, F.; Fitchet, M. A Randomized Double-Blind Placebo-Controlled Study of the Long-Term Efficacy and Safety of Topiramate in the Treatment of Obese Subjects. *Int. J. Obes. Relat. Metab. Disord.* **2004**, *28*, 1399–1410. [CrossRef] [PubMed]
14. Toplak, H.; Hamann, A.; Moore, R.; Masson, E.; Gorska, M.; Vercruysse, F.; Sun, X.; Fitchet, M. Efficacy and Safety of Topiramate in Combination with Metformin in the Treatment of Obese Subjects with Type 2 Diabetes: A Randomized, Double-Blind, Placebo-Controlled Study. *Int. J. Obes.* **2007**, *31*, 138–146. [CrossRef] [PubMed]
15. Eliasson, B.; Gudbjörnsdottir, S.; Cederholm, J.; Liang, Y.; Vercruysse, F.; Smith, U. Weight Loss and Metabolic Effects of Topiramate in Overweight and Obese Type 2 Diabetic Patients: Randomized Double-Blind Placebo-Controlled Trial. *Int. J. Obes.* **2007**, *31*, 1140–1147. [CrossRef]
16. El-Abhar, H.S.; Schaalan, M.F. Topiramate-Induced Modulation of Hepatic Molecular Mechanisms: An Aspect for Its Anti-Insulin Resistant Effect. *PLoS ONE* **2012**, *7*, e37757. [CrossRef]
17. Wahjudi, P.N.; Lu, Q.-Y.; Patterson, M.E.; Zhang, X.; Go, V.L.; Chen, J.; Li, W.-L.; Lee, W.N.P. Anti-Hyperglycemic Effect of Loquat Leaf Extract Is Associated with the Redistribution of Glucose Carbon to Its Metabolites: A 13c-Tracing Study in Hepg2 Cells. *Metabolomics* **2017**, *13*, 91. [CrossRef]
18. Lu, Q.Y.; Zhang, L.; Yee, J.K.; Go, V.W.; Lee, W.N. Metabolic Consequences of Ldha Inhibition by Epigallocatechin Gallate and Oxamate in Mia Paca-2 Pancreatic Cancer Cells. *Metabolomics* **2015**, *11*, 71–80. [CrossRef]
19. Lu, Q.; Summanen, P.H.; Lee, R.; Huang, J.; Henning, S.M.; Heber, D.; Finegold, S.M.; Li, Z. Prebiotic Potential and Chemical Composition of Seven Culinary Spice Extracts. *J. Food Sci.* **2017**, *82*, 1807–1813. [CrossRef]
20. Buescher, J.M.; Antoniewicz, M.R.; Boros, L.G.; Burgess, S.C.; Brunengraber, H.; Clish, C.B.; DeBerardinis, R.J.; Feron, O.; Frezza, C.; Ghesquiere, B.; et al. A roadmap for interpreting ^{13}C metabolite labeling patterns from cells. *Curr. Opin. Biotechnol.* **2015**, *34*, 189–201. [CrossRef]
21. Rebello, C.J.; Beyl, R.A.; Lertora, J.J.; Greenway, F.L.; Ravussin, E.; Ribnicky, D.M.; Poulev, A.; Kennedy, B.J.; Castro, H.F.; Campagna, S.R.; et al. Safety and Pharmacokinetics of Naringenin: A Randomized, Controlled, Single-Ascending-Dose Clinical Trial. *Diabetes Obes. Metab.* **2020**, *22*, 91–98. [CrossRef] [PubMed]
22. Xiao, B.; Jiang, Y.; Yuan, S.; Cai, L.; Xu, T.; Jia, L. Silibinin, a Potential Fasting Mimetic, Inhibits Hepatocellular Carcinoma by Triggering Extrinsic Apoptosis. *MedComm* **2024**, *5*, e457. [CrossRef] [PubMed]
23. Wilkes, J.J.; Nelson, E.; Osborne, M.; Demarest, K.T.; Olefsky, J.M. Topiramate Is an Insulin-Sensitizing Compound in Vivo with Direct Effects on Adipocytes in Female Zdf Rats. *Am. J. Physiol. Endocrinol. Metab.* **2005**, *288*, E617–E624. [CrossRef] [PubMed]
24. Allende, D.S.; Gawrieh, S.; Cummings, O.W.; Belt, P.; Wilson, L.; Van Natta, M.; Behling, C.A.; Carpenter, D.; Gill, R.M.; Kleiner, D.E.; et al. Glycogenosis is common in nonalcoholic fatty liver disease and is independently associated with ballooning, but lower steatosis and lower fibrosis. *Liver Int.* **2021**, *41*, 996–1011. [CrossRef] [PubMed]
25. Marin, S.; Lee, W.N.; Bassilian, S.; Lim, S.; Boros, L.G.; Centelles, J.J.; FernAndez-Novell, J.M.; Guinovart, J.J.; Cascante, M. Dynamic profiling of the glucose metabolic network in fasted rat hepatocytes using [1,2-13C2]glucose. *Biochem. J.* **2004**, *381 Pt 1*, 287–294. [CrossRef]
26. Lee, W.N.; Byerley, L.O.; Bergner, E.A.; Edmond, J. Mass Isotopomer Analysis: Theoretical and Practical Considerations. *Biol. Mass. Spectrom.* **1991**, *20*, 451–458. [CrossRef]

27. Jia, Y.; Yee, J.K.; Wang, C.; Nikolaenko, L.; Diaz-Arjonilla, M.; Cohen, J.N.; French, S.W.; Liu, P.Y.; Lue, Y.; Lee, W.N.; et al. Testosterone protects high-fat/low-carbohydrate diet-induced nonalcoholic fatty liver disease in castrated male rats mainly via modulating endoplasmic reticulum stress. *Am. J. Physiol. Endocrinol. Metab.* **2018**, *314*, E366–E376. [CrossRef]
28. Boros, L.G.; Deng, Q.; Pandol, S.J.; Tsukamoto, H.; Go, V.L.; Lee, W.N. Ethanol diversely alters palmitate, stearate, and oleate metabolism in the liver and pancreas of rats using the deuterium oxide single tracer. *Pancreas* **2009**, *38*, e47–e52. [CrossRef]
29. Lee, W.N.; Edmond, J.; Bassilian, S.; Morrow, J.W. Mass Isotopomer Study of Glutamine Oxidation and Synthesis in Primary Culture of Astrocytes. *Dev. Neurosci.* **1996**, *18*, 469–477. [CrossRef]
30. Leimer, K.R.; Rice, R.H.; Gehrke, C.W. Complete Mass Spectra of N-Trifluoroacetyl-N-Butyl Esters of Amino Acids. *J. Chromatogr.* **1977**, *141*, 121–144. [CrossRef]
31. Lee, W.N.; Boros, L.G.; Puigjaner, J.; Bassilian, S.; Lim, S.; Cascante, M. Mass Isotopomer Study of the Nonoxidative Pathways of the Pentose Cycle with [1,2-13c2]Glucose. *Am. J. Physiol.* **1998**, *274*, E843–E851. [CrossRef]
32. Araya, J.; Rodrigo, R.; Videla, L.A.; Thielemann, L.; Orellana, M.; Pettinelli, P.; Poniachik, J. Increase in Long-Chain Polyunsaturated Fatty Acid $N-6/N-3$ Ratio in Relation to Hepatic Steatosis in Patients with Non-Alcoholic Fatty Liver Disease. *Clin. Sci.* **2004**, *106*, 635–643. [CrossRef]
33. Ricchi, M.; Odoardi, M.R.; Carulli, L.; Anzivino, C.; Ballestri, S.; Pinetti, A.; Fantoni, L.I.; Marra, F.; Bertolotti, M.; Banni, S.; et al. Differential Effect of Oleic and Palmitic Acid on Lipid Accumulation and Apoptosis in Cultured Hepatocytes. *J. Gastroenterol. Hepatol.* **2009**, *24*, 830–840. [CrossRef]
34. Rafiei, H.; Omidian, K.; Bandy, B. Comparison of Dietary Polyphenols for Protection against Molecular Mechanisms Underlying Nonalcoholic Fatty Liver Disease in a Cell Model of Steatosis. *Mol. Nutr. Food Res.* **2017**, *61*, 9. [CrossRef]
35. Liu, Y.; Liao, L.; Chen, Y.; Han, F. Effects of Daphnetin on Lipid Metabolism, Insulin Resistance and Oxidative Stress in Oa-Treated Hepg2 Cells. *Mol. Med. Rep.* **2019**, *19*, 4673–4684. [CrossRef]
36. Go, Y.; Jeong, J.Y.; Jeoung, N.H.; Jeon, J.-H.; Park, B.-Y.; Kang, H.-J.; Ha, C.-M.; Choi, Y.-K.; Lee, S.J.; Ham, H.J.; et al. Inhibition of Pyruvate Dehydrogenase Kinase 2 Protects Against Hepatic Steatosis Through Modulation of Tricarboxylic Acid Cycle Anaplerosis and Ketogenesis. *Diabetes* **2016**, *65*, 2876–2887. [CrossRef]
37. Fletcher, J.A.; Deja, S.; Satapati, S.; Fu, X.; Burgess, S.C.; Browning, J.D. Impaired ketogenesis and increased acetyl-CoA oxidation promote hyperglycemia in human fatty liver. *JCI Insight* **2019**, *5*, e127737. [CrossRef]
38. Harris, D.M.; Li, L.; Chen, M.; Lagunero, F.T.; Go, V.L.; Boros, L.G. Diverse Mechanisms of Growth Inhibition by Luteolin, Resveratrol, and Quercetin in Mia Paca-2 Cells: A Comparative Glucose Tracer Study with the Fatty Acid Synthase Inhibitor C75. *Metabolomics* **2012**, *8*, 201–210. [CrossRef]
39. Liu, Y.; Xu, W.; Zhai, T.; You, J.; Chen, Y. Silibinin Ameliorates Hepatic Lipid Accumulation and Oxidative Stress in Mice with Non-Alcoholic Steatohepatitis by Regulating Cflar-Jnk Pathway. *Acta Pharm. Sin. B* **2019**, *9*, 745–757. [CrossRef]
40. Kapoor, R.; Kakkar, P. Protective role of morin, a flavonoid, against high glucose induced oxidative stress mediated apoptosis in primary rat hepatocytes. *PLoS ONE* **2012**, *7*, e41663. [CrossRef]
41. Wang, Q.; Ou, Y.; Hu, G.; Wen, C.; Yue, S.; Chen, C.; Xu, L.; Xie, J.; Dai, H.; Xiao, H.; et al. Naringenin attenuates non-alcoholic fatty liver disease by down-regulating the NLRP3/NF-κB pathway in mice. *Br. J. Pharmacol.* **2020**, *177*, 1806–1821. [CrossRef] [PubMed]

nutrients

MDPI

Article

Preliminary Data on the Senolytic Effects of *Agrimonia pilosa* Ledeb. Extract Containing Agrimols for Immunosenescence in Middle-Aged Humans: A Randomized, Double-Blind, Placebo-Controlled, Parallel-Group Comparison Study

Yoshiki Shimizu [1,*], Shieri Shimodan [1], Mariko Hayashida [1], Misato Yazaki [1], Tsuyoshi Sakurada [1], Tomomichi Watanabe [1], Yuri Ishii [1], Yoshie Hirose [2], Jiro Saito [3] and Sachiyuki Teramoto [1]

[1] FANCL Research Institute, FANCL Corporation, 12-13 Kamishinano, Totsuka-ku, Yokohama 244-0806, Japan; shieri2104@fancl.co.jp (S.S.); mariko1512@fancl.co.jp (M.H.); misato_110401@fancl.co.jp (M.Y.); sakurada_tsuyoshi@fancl.co.jp (T.S.); watanabe_tomomichi@fancl.co.jp (T.W.); yuishii@fancl.co.jp (Y.I.); sateramoto@fancl.co.jp (S.T.)

[2] Yukeikai Medical Corporation Ginza Yoshie Clinic, V88 Building 5F, 2-5-11 Ginza, Chuo-ku, Tokyo 104-0061, Japan; yh@ginzabiyou.com

[3] Medical Station Clinic, 3F Ichikawa Gakugei-dai Building, 3-12-8 Takaban, Meguro-ku, Tokyo 152-0004, Japan; j.saito@med-station.jp

* Correspondence: shimizu_yoshiki@fancl.co.jp; Tel.: +81-45-820-3755

Abstract: Objectives: To assess the effects of agrimol-containing *Agrimonia pilosa* Ledeb. extract (APE) for senescent immune cell removal in middle-aged Japanese adults with immunosenescence. Design and Setting: A randomized, double-blind, placebo-controlled, parallel-group study was conducted in Japan between June 2023 and April 2024. Participants: 110 individuals aged 40–59, selected based on CD8+ T cells with highly-expressing-senescence-associated-β-galactosidase (SA-βGal). Intervention: Participants were randomly assigned to receive 50 mg APE containing 0.2 mg of agrimols or a placebo for eight consecutive weeks. Measurements: The primary endpoint was the change in the proportion of CD8+ T cells with high SA-βGal expression at 8 weeks of intake from the baseline. The secondary endpoints included the proportion of CD4+ T cells with high SA-βGal expression, CD4+ and CD8+ T cell subsets, and the ratio of various immune cells. Results: Of the 635 subjects screened, 110 with immunosenescence were included in this study. In total, 55 participants in the placebo group and 53 in the APE group completed the intervention. There were no statistically significant changes in either the primary or secondary endpoints due to APE intake. In the male population, the proportion of CD8+ T cells with high SA-βGal expression was reduced by APE intake ($p = 0.044$). Furthermore, the proportion of naïve CD8+ T cells increased and the number of effector memory CD8+ T cells decreased with the consumption of APE. Conclusions: APE was suggested to reduce senescent immune cells, indicating its potential as a candidate senolytic agent for humans; however, the results of this study are preliminary data, and further research on APE is needed (clinical trial registration: UMIN000051574).

Keywords: *Agrimonia pilosa* Ledeb. extract; agrimol; immunosenescence; senolytic agent; senescence-associated β-galactosidase

1. Introduction

In recent years, the global population has been growing older, and it is estimated that the proportion of the world's elderly aged 65 years or older will reach 16% by 2050, compared to approximately 10% in 2022 [1]. While the average lifespan is increasing, the number of elderly people with physical, mental, and social problems due to the aging process is also increasing, as is the risk of death and the need for nursing care for the elderly [2–4]. Aging, or senescence, is a process that typically begins around the age of 40 and is driven by genetic and environmental factors that cause a gradual decline in physiological functions [5–7].

Senescence is defined as an irreversible pathophysiological process involving the progressive decline of mental and physical functions in postmature organisms [5,6]. Cellular senescence, a key hallmark of aging, is a state in which cells cease to proliferate irreversibly due to various stressors and plays an important role in suppressing tumorigenesis, wound healing, and tissue repair [8]. Although senescent cells provide these beneficial functions, their accumulation leads to tissue dysfunction and chronic inflammation through the senescence-associated secretory phenotype (SASP), which contributes to various aging-related diseases [9,10]. Therapeutic strategies targeting senescent cells, such as senolytic agents, have shown promise in animal models. Senolytic agents selectively remove senescent cells, alleviating age-related disorders and extending lifespan by reducing the secretion of SASP factors [7,11–14]. These findings underscore the importance of further investigating senolytic therapies as a means of mitigating the negative effects of aging.

One of the key manifestations of aging is immunosenescence, which refers to the age-related decline in immune function. Immunosenescence is characterized by thymic atrophy, a decrease in the proportion of naïve T cells, an increase in memory T cells, and heightened chronic inflammation [15]. These changes are hallmarks of immunosenescence and increase the risk of infection and other diseases in elderly individuals [16,17]. Animal studies highlight the harmful effects of immunosenescence, such as accelerated aging and reduced lifespan due to mitochondrial dysfunction in T cells [18]. Perforin-knockout mice with deficient immune surveillance accumulate more senescent cells with age compared to control mice. These mice develop multiple age-related diseases and have a reduced survival rate [19]. In other words, the accumulation of senescent immune cells during immunosenescence may be a risk factor not only for disease but also for aging.

Among senescence markers, senescence-associated β-galactosidase (SA-βGal) is widely used due to its high expression in senescent cells. While not its optimal pH, SA-βGal activity can be detected at pH 6.0 and serves as an indicator of increased lysosomal mass in senescent cells [20–22]. Martínez-Zamudio et al. demonstrated the utility of fluorescence-activated cell sorting (FACS) technology in identifying senescent immune cells. Their study showed that older adults have a higher proportion of high-SA-βGal-expressing CD8+ T cells, which are characterized by telomere dysfunction, elevated p16 expression, and p16-induced senescence [23].

In our research group, we utilized FACS to sort peripheral blood CD8+ T cells into high- and low-SA-βGal-expressing cell populations and performed preliminary analysis (unpublished data). The results showed that high-SA-βGal-expressing CD8+ T cells displayed significantly higher p16 expression compared to low-SA-βGal CD8+ T cells, with the observations reported by Martínez-Zamudio et al. [23]. These findings suggest that SA-βGal is a reliable marker of senescence. In other words, measuring SA-βGal expression in peripheral blood CD8+ T cells allows for a minimally invasive evaluation of senolytic therapies for immunosenescence.

Agrimonia pilosa Ledeb., also known as Pilosa Cocklebur, is a plant of the family Rosaceae traditionally used in Chinese medicine. It contains many bioactive compounds, such as phloroglucinols, flavonoids, tannins, phenols, triterpenoids, and organic acids [24–26]. *A. pilosa* Ledeb. extract (APE) has been reported to have medicinal effects, such as antioxidant, anti-inflammatory, antibacterial, antitumor, and anti-diabetic effects, and is attracting attention as a food material with anti-aging effects [27–31]. APE and agrimol B, a phloroglucinol derived from *A. pilosa* Ledeb., have been shown to induce apoptosis in doxorubicin-induced senescent cells and reduce senescence markers such as p16 and SASP factors in aged mice [32]. Watanabe et al. reported that APE administration in aged mice led to a reduction in high-SA-βGal CD8+ T cells and a decrease in memory CD8+ T cells and promoted an increase in naïve CD8+ T cells, suggesting its potential to alleviate immunosenescence [32]. These findings indicate that APE may mitigate immunosenescence, making it a promising candidate as a senolytic agent.

However, the senolytic effects of APE in humans remain unclear. Therefore, we conducted a randomized, double-blind, placebo-controlled parallel-group comparison study to obtain preliminary data on the senolytic effects of APE-containing agrimols on senescent immune cells in middle-aged Japanese men and women with immunosenescence using FACS technology with SA-βGal as a marker. We also investigated potential sex differences in the effects of APE.

2. Materials and Methods

2.1. Study Setting

This study was reviewed and approved (approval date: 22 June 2023; review number: 230622-1; principal investigators: Sayuri Matsuoka [until 30 September 2023] and Sachiyuki Teramoto [from 1 October 2023]) by the Medical Station Clinic Ethics Review Committee, which is composed of unrelated third parties (IRB number: 20000022). This study was conducted following the Declaration of Helsinki (revised in October 2013) and in accordance with the Ethical Guidelines for Medical and Health Research Involving Human Subjects (Notification No. 1 by the Ministry of Education, Culture, Sports, Science and Technology; Ministry of Health, Labour and Welfare; and Ministry of Economy, Trade and Industry; 23 March 2021 [partially revised on 27 March 2023]) and the Guidance for Ethical Guidelines for Medical and Health Research Involving Human Subjects (Ministry of Education, Culture, Sports, Science and Technology; Ministry of Health, Labour and Welfare; and Ministry of Economy, Trade and Industry; 16 April 2021 [partially revised on 17 April 2023]). Before this study, the principal investigational doctor thoroughly explained the purpose and details of the study to the participants. Written informed consent was obtained from all participants, and only those who provided consent were included.

This study was conducted using the participant management and research implementation systems provided by the Medical Station Clinic and Yukeikai Medical Corporation Ginza Yoshie Clinic. The principal investigational doctor (Jiro Saito) and one of the investigational doctors (Yoshie Hirose) supervised all research-related activities, including providing instructions to the participants of this study, obtaining consent, conducting interviews, and managing the examination system. The principal investigational doctor confirmed and assessed the adverse events, prepared case reports, and administered the necessary treatments for adverse events, as needed. This study was conducted between June 2023 and April 2024. Prior to the commencement of the trial, the study details were registered with the University Hospital Medical Information Network Clinical Trials Registry (UMIN-CTR) (clinical trial registration: UMIN000051574).

2.2. Subjects

Subject characteristics such as medical history, drinking and eating habits, clinical and physical examinations, and peripheral blood mononuclear cell (PBMC) tests were conducted to screen 635 participants, whose consent was obtained in writing prior to study participation. Based on the screening test results, 110 participants who met the selection criteria and did not meet the exclusion criteria were selected. Participants were enrolled in order of the proportion of their high-SA-βGal-expressing CD8+ T cells (high-SA-βGal CD8+ T cells) from among the group of prospective participants.

Participants were selected based on the following criteria: Japanese male and female participants aged 40–59 years at the time of obtaining consent, participants with a relatively high proportion of high-SA-βGal CD8+ T cells, subjects who could provide consent, and those who did not meet the exclusion criteria. The exclusion criteria were participants who had undergone surgical resection of the gastrointestinal tract (not including appendectomy); participants who had a disease that required constant medication or those with a serious medical history that required medication; participants with autoimmune diseases or a history of autoimmune diseases; participants with mental illness, chronic fatigue syndrome, insomnia, or a history of such illnesses; patients diagnosed with or suspected of having sleep apnea; participants undergoing treatment related to sleep, stress, and/or fatigue; night-and-day-shift workers or manual laborers; participants who regularly took or planned to take medicines, supplements, Foods for Specified Health Uses (FOSHU), and/or foods that may have affected the results during the study; participants with possibilities of emerging allergies related to the study intervention; heavy drinkers and excessive smokers; participants who were planning to travel abroad during the study period or who were planning a long-term domestic trip for more than one week in the study period; participants who were judged unsuitable for the study based on the results of the lifestyle questionnaire; participants who were judged unsuitable for the study based on the results of their clinical laboratory or cardiopulmonary function tests; participants whose physical measurements, physical examination values, and clinical examination values before the start of intake were significantly outside the reference range; participants who were participating in other clinical studies at the start of the study; participants who were pregnant or intended to become pregnant; and participants whom the investigator judged as unsuitable for the study for other reasons.

2.3. *Sample Size Calculation*

Based on data from a previous study using APE (UMIN000048415), we calculated that a sample size of 55 participants per group (totaling 110 subjects) would be necessary for this study. This calculation accounted for an anticipated difference of 4.6% in the change in the proportion of high-SA-βGal CD8+ T cells between the APE group and the placebo group, with a common standard deviation of 8.1%. This study assumed a two-sided significance level of 5% and a power of 0.8 for the Student's *t*-test, considering potential dropout cases during the trial or exclusions due to protocol violations.

2.4. *Trial Intervention*

The APE used in this study was prepared by Maruzen Pharmaceuticals Co., Ltd. (Hiroshima, Japan) from dried *A. pilosa* Ledeb. The extraction process involved using aqueous ethanol to extract the active components, removing water-soluble substances, concentrating hydrophobic components containing agrimols, and then drying and pulverizing them with excipients. The specification for the APE ensured that it contained at least 0.4% agrimols.

The test food consisted of hard capsules containing 50 mg APE per capsule. Each 50 mg of APE contained 0.2 mg of agrimols, including agrimol B. The placebo capsules were identical in appearance to the test food capsules. They contained cellulose instead of APE and were colored similarly to ensure indistinguishability from the test food. The test food was administered to the subjects in the form of one capsule (50 mg APE or placebo) per day, taken with water or warm water.

In studies evaluating the effects of immunosenescence, interventions are sometimes conducted over a period of approximately four to eight weeks [33–36]. Additionally, from our research group's previous study involving APE intake (UMIN000048415), it was considered that the intervention effects of APE could be observed within about eight weeks. Therefore, the intake period for the study food in this research was set to eight weeks (56 days).

2.5. Trial Protocol

This was a randomized, double-blind, placebo-controlled, parallel-group comparison study. The randomization of participants into the APE and placebo groups was performed by Yoshihisa Kibune (Consultant, EP Mediate Co., Ltd., Tokyo, Japan) using computer-generated random numbers based on the participants selected during screening. Blinding was applied to all parties involved in this study (participants, intervention administrators, and evaluators), and the code was not broken until the analysis population was fixed.

After randomization, the subjects were brought in for baseline tests, which included weight measurement, blood pressure and pulse measurement, blood sampling (for peripheral blood mononuclear cells [PBMCs] and serum), urine collection, medical interviews, and questionnaire surveys. Subjects who completed the baseline examinations were administered APE or the placebo and began their intake. Starting from the first day of intake, participants returned for follow-up visits at 4 and 8 weeks, where they underwent weight measurement, blood pressure and pulse measurement, blood sampling (for PBMC and serum), urine collection, medical interviews, and questionnaire surveys. The specified examination days for the 4-week and 8-week assessments were set as days 29 and 57, respectively, and the baseline examination was counted as day 1. However, the principal investigational doctor could reschedule the examinations within seven days before or after the specified examination days if necessary. During the intake period, participants were asked to record their intake of trial supplements, exercise, alcohol consumption, physical condition, and use of medications.

The investigational doctors instructed the subjects not to change their lifestyle habits from the time of consent until the end of the intervention period. If any changes in the subjects' lifestyle habits were observed in their records, the investigational doctors provided guidance to ensure that the subjects maintained their original lifestyle habits.

Blood tests included counts and measurements of white blood cells, red blood cells, hemoglobin, hematocrit, MCV, MCH, MCHC, platelets, total protein (TP), albumin (Alb), A/G ratio, total bilirubin (TB), direct bilirubin (D-B), indirect bilirubin (I-B), ALP at screening and at 8 weeks of intake, AST (GOT), ALT (GPT), LD, γGT (γGTP), total cholesterol (TC), triglycerides (TG), HDL cholesterol (HDL-C), LDL cholesterol (LDL-C), urea nitrogen (UN), creatinine (Cr), uric acid (UA), Na, K, Cl, blood sugar (GLU), HbA1c, insulin, Fe, total iron binding capacity (TIBC), unsaturated iron binding capacity (UIBC), and cystatin C. Urinalysis was performed for protein (qualitative), sugar (qualitative), and occult blood reaction (qualitative). Blood tests and urinalyses were performed by LSI Medience Corporation (Tokyo, Japan) using a standardized method.

2.6. Peripheral Blood Mononuclear Cell (PBMC) Collection and Preservation

To collect PBMCs, blood was drawn from participants using BD Vacutainer® CPT™ Mononuclear Cell Preparation Tubes with Sodium Citrate (BD Biosciences, Franklin Lakes, NJ, USA). Blood was drawn for PBMC collection in 8 mL volumes on each test day. After blood collection, the samples were centrifuged to isolate PBMCs. The PBMC layer was then collected into 15 mL tubes, resuspended in PBS(-) (Thermo Fisher Scientific, Inc., Waltham, MA, USA), and centrifuged again. After removing the supernatant, the cells were resuspended in Bambanker® medium (NIPPON Genetics Co., Ltd., Tokyo, Japan) and stored at −80 °C until use.

2.7. Flow Cytometric Analyses

Cell staining was performed as previously described, with some modifications [23]. Bafilomycin A1 and SPiDER-βGal included in the Cellular Senescence Detection Kit-SPiDER-βGal (Dojindo Laboratories, Kumamoto, Japan) were dissolved in 30 μL and 20 μL of dimethyl sulfoxide (FUJIFILM Wako Pure Chemical Corporation, Osaka, Japan), respectively. After thawing cryopreserved 5×10^5 human PBMCs and washing them with FACS Buffer (PBS(-), 2% FBS (*v*/*v*) (Thermo Fisher Scientific, Inc.), 2 mM EDTA (Thermo Fisher Scientific, Inc.) and 1% penicillin-streptomycin (Sigma Aldrich, St. Louis, MO, USA)), the PBMCs were treated with bafilomycin A1 diluted 1:500 in HBSS(-) (FUJIFILM Wako Pure Chemical Corporation) at 37 °C for 1.5 h. In addition to SA-βGal, endogenous βGal was also present in the cells and was expressed regardless of senescence. SPiDER-βGal reacted with both βGals, but with bafilomycin A1 treatment, which inhibited only endogenous βGal, only SA-βGal was specifically detected.

The PBMCs were treated with both SPiDER-βGal and bafilomycin A1 (diluted 1:500 in HBSS(-)) at 37 °C for another 30 min. After washing with FACS Buffer, the PBMCs were treated with human TruStain FcX™ (Biolegend, San Diego, CA, USA, diluted 1:100) on ice for 20 min. After treatment with PE-conjugated anti-human CD3 antibody (SK7, 1:100), Brilliant Violet 510™-conjugated anti-human CD4 antibody (SK3, 1:100), PerCP/Cyanine5.5-conjugated anti-human CD8a antibody (RPA-T8, 1:100), Alexa Fluor® 647-conjugated anti human CD45RA antibody (HI100, 1:5000), Brilliant Violet 421™-conjugated anti-human CD197 antibody (CCR7) (G043H7, 3:100), and PE/Cyanine7-conjugated anti-human CD279 (PD-1) antibody (EH12.2H7, 1:100) (all from Biolegend, San Diego, CA, USA), the PBMCs were incubated on ice for 30 min. The PBMCs, which were stained for SA-βGal using the same procedure as described above, were also treated with Alexa Fluor®647-conjugated Mouse IgG2b, k Isotype Ctrl (MPC-11, 1:50000), Brilliant Violet 421™-conjugated Mouse IgG2a, k Isotype Ctrl (MOPC-173, 21:500), PE/Cyanine7-conjugated Mouse IgG1, and k Isotype Ctrl (MOPC-21, 1:100) (all from Biolegend), used as isotype controls. After washing the antibody-stained PBMCs with FACS Buffer, the PBMCs were treated with Fixable Viability Dye eFluor™ 780 (Thermo Fisher Scientific, Inc., 1:1000) on ice for 20 min. The stained PBMCs were analyzed using a BD FACS Celesta instrument (BD Biosciences) and FlowJo software v10.8.1 (FlowJo, LLC, Ashland, OR, USA). The PBMCs for flow cytometric analysis were acquired at 100,000 events. Each subset of CD4+ and CD8+ T cells was identified using the following markers based on the isotype controls:

- Naïve T cells: CD197(CCR7)+CD45RA+
- Central memory T cells: CD197(CCR7)+CD45RA-
- Effector memory T cells: CD197(CCR7)-CD45RA-
- Terminally differentiated effector memory T cells re-expressing CD45RA (TEMRA): CD197(CCR7)-CD45RA+
- PD-1-positive cells: CD279+

To quantify the percentage of T cells expressing high levels of SA-βGal, we took advantage of the fact that donors often had separate populations consisting of cells with low and high SA-βGal fluorescence. Specifically, we set a gate at the intersection of the two populations; the high population with low signal intensity was designated as "SA-βGal low" and the population with high signal intensity was designated as "SA-βGal high".

2.8. Digital PCR for Gene Expression of Cell Cycle Markers and Sirt1 in PBMCs

Digital PCR (dPCR) was conducted to assess the gene expression levels of cell cycle markers (p16, p21, p53) and Sirtuin 1 (Sirt1).

Total RNA was extracted and purified from 1×10^6 PBMCs using the RNeasy 96 Kit (QIAGEN, Venlo, The Netherlands) according to the manufacturer's instructions. cDNA was synthesized from purified total RNA by reverse transcription using a PrimeScript™ RT Reagent kit (Takara Bio, Inc., Shiga, Japan).

Absolute quantification of RNA levels was conducted using QIAcuity digital PCR (QIAGEN, Venlo, The Netherlands) with the QIAcuity Nanoplate 8.5 K 96-well (QIAGEN). dPCR was performed with TaqMan probes (Applied Biosystems, Foster City, CA, USA) targeting the following genes: *Actb* (assay ID: Hs01060665_g1), *CDKN2A* (Hs00923894_m1), *CDKN1A* (Hs00355782_m1), *TP53* (Hs01034249_m1), and *Sirt1* (Hs01009006_m1). For each well, 12 μL of reaction solution was prepared, including 3 μL of 4x Probe PCR Master Mix (Takara Bio Inc., Shiga, Japan), 0.4 μM TaqMan Probe, and cDNA template. The thermal cycling program consisted of 20 s at 95 °C, 45 cycles of 1 s at 95 °C, and 20 s at 60 °C. The fraction of target gene for each sample was determined by dividing the number of copies/μL of the target gene by the number of copies/μL of the *Actb* gene. Samples with insufficient template RNA or issues with the accuracy of measurement results were treated as missing values.

2.9. Outcome Measures

2.9.1. Efficacy Evaluation

The primary endpoint of this study was the change in the proportion of high-SA-βGal CD8+ T cells in human PBMCs from baseline to week 8.

The secondary endpoints of this study included changes from baseline to week 8 in the following parameters: the proportion of high-SA-βGal CD4+ T cells in human PBMCs; the proportion of naïve cells, central memory cells, effector memory cells, TEMRA cells, and PD-1 expressing cells among both CD8+ and CD4+ T cells in human PBMCs; and the ratios of CD3+ T cells/lymphocytes, CD4+ T cells/lymphocytes, CD8+ T cells/lymphocytes, and CD4+/CD8+ T cells in human PBMCs.

In addition, as a subgroup analysis specified in the study protocol, efficacy evaluations were conducted according to sex.

2.9.2. Exploratory Efficacy Evaluation

As an assessment of senescence markers other than SA-βGal, the expression levels of p16, p21, p53, and Sirt1 in the PBMC population were evaluated.

2.9.3. Safety Evaluation

Safety was assessed by evaluating the test values of each examination item at week 8 and any adverse events that occurred after the intake of the trial supplements.

2.10. Statistical Analysis

The APE and placebo groups for each item were evaluated using Student's *t*-test. Analysis of covariance (ANCOVA) was performed using the baseline values as covariates when necessary, such as when differences in baseline values were found between groups. The screening data for enrolled subjects and those who were not included in this study were compared using Student's *t*-test. The baseline characteristics of the placebo and APE groups were compared using either Student's *t*-test or Fisher's exact test. The values for each test and evaluation item were presented as the mean ± standard deviation or the mean ± standard error. The significance level for the tests was set at 5% (two-sided). Statistical analyses were performed using IBM SPSS Statistics 29 software (International Business Machines Corporation, Armonk, NY, USA) and JMP® 17 software (SAS Institute Inc., Cary, NC, USA).

3. Results

3.1. Characteristics of the Study Subjects

Screening tests were performed on 635 potential candidates for whom consent was obtained, and 110 subjects were selected. All 110 selected subjects were randomly assigned to the placebo group (N = 55; male, 28; female, 27) or the test food group (N = 55; male, 27; female, 28). A comparison of the screening test endpoints for the enrolled and non-enrolled participants is shown in Table 1. While there was no significant difference in age between the groups, the enrolled participants had a significantly higher proportion of high-SA-βGal CD8+ and CD4+ T cells compared to the non-enrolled group. This suggested that the enrolled subjects represented a cohort with immunosenescence within the 40–50-year-old age range. Additionally, the number of naïve T cells, which typically decrease with age, was significantly lower in the enrolled participants, whereas the numbers of effector memory and TEMRA cells were significantly higher. Furthermore, the proportion of PD-1-positive cells, a marker of exhausted T cells, was significantly higher in the enrolled subjects than in the non-enrolled group. These findings indicated that the enrolled subjects had more advanced immunosenescence relative to their age based on their T cell subset populations.

Table 1. Comparison of the population of T cells and their subsets and immunosenescence markers between enrolled and non-enrolled subjects.

		Overall		Non-Enrolled		Enrolled		
		N = 632		N = 522		N = 110		
Items		Mean	SD	Mean	SD	Mean	SD	*p* Value
	Age (years)	50.2	5.2	50.2	5.3	50.0	4.9	0.6057
CD8+	High SA-βGal (%)	65.46	20.07	61.05	19.26	86.36	5.08	<0.0001
	Naïve (%)	34.56	17.50	38.29	16.79	16.86	6.56	<0.0001
	Central memory (%)	21.51	9.37	21.91	9.29	19.59	9.57	0.0182
	Effector memory (%)	30.09	12.52	27.93	11.64	40.31	11.48	<0.0001
	TEMRA (%)	13.85	11.69	11.87	10.12	23.24	13.93	<0.0001
	PD-1+ (%)	9.815	5.834	9.710	5.640	10.312	6.685	0.3255
CD4+	High SA-βGal (%)	52.32	17.78	49.94	17.36	63.62	15.27	<0.0001
	Naïve (%)	19.94	10.07	20.97	10.07	15.04	8.52	<0.0001
	Central memory (%)	62.93	9.56	62.79	9.58	63.63	9.49	0.3987
	Effector memory (%)	16.78	7.74	15.95	7.41	20.73	8.09	<0.0001
	TEMRA (%)	0.348	0.800	0.297	0.673	0.593	1.210	0.0004
	PD-1+ (%)	12.407	4.948	12.124	4.995	13.747	4.507	0.0017
CD3+/Lymphocyte (%)		78.01	8.41	77.86	8.53	78.71	7.81	0.3379
CD4+/Lymphocyte (%)		52.94	8.74	53.45	8.70	50.47	8.57	0.0011
CD8+/Lymphocyte (%)		19.12	6.59	18.68	6.37	21.23	7.19	0.0002
CD4+/CD8+		3.20	1.51	3.30	1.53	2.76	1.30	0.0007

Values are represented as means ± SDs. "Overall" is the total subject population for which consent was obtained, "Non-enrolled" is the population that was deemed ineligible for participation or withdrew consent during screening or testing, and "Enrolled" is the population of subjects who were enrolled. Student's *t*-test was used to compare Enrolled and Non-enrolled.

Of the 110 enrolled subjects, one subject in the APE group withdrew consent to participate in the study before attending the baseline examination and another subject in the food group began taking the test supplement but did not attend the baseline or 4-week examination. The principal investigational doctor determined that it would be difficult for the participants to continue in this study and subsequently terminated their participation. Finally, a total of 108 subjects completed the prescribed study schedule: 55 in the placebo group and 53 in the APE group (Figure 1).

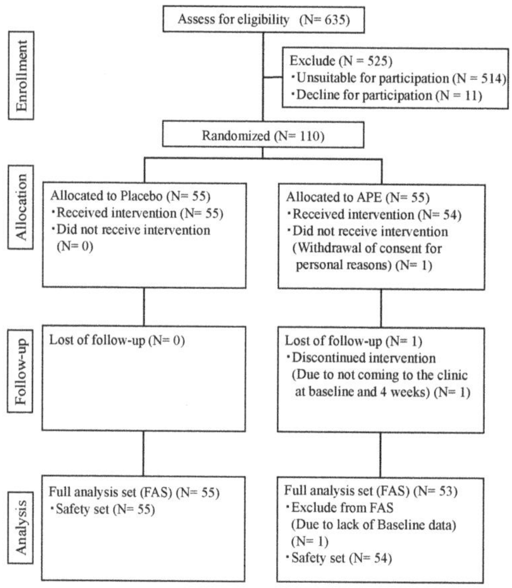

Figure 1. Participant flow.

Of the 108 patients who completed the study schedule, one (placebo group) had an 89.3% intake rate of the trial supplement, one (placebo group) had a 96.4% intake rate, four (two in the placebo group and two in the APE group) had a 98.2% intake rate, and the remaining 102 had a 100% intake rate. The average intake rates were 99.7% for the placebo group and 99.97% for the APE group. Of the 110 patients allocated to the trial supplement, 108 with data on primary and secondary endpoints after baseline testing were included in the full analysis set (FAS), representing the largest analysis population. The safety set consisted of 109 patients (55 in the placebo group and 54 in the test food group), excluding one patient in the test food group who did not start taking the trial supplement.

As baseline characteristics for the FAS, Table 2 shows the results for age, height, weight, body mass index, systolic blood pressure, diastolic blood pressure, pulse rate, proportion of high = SA-βGal CD8+ and CD4+ T cells, T cell subsets, proportion of PD-1-expressing cells, and proportions of CD3+, CD4+, and CD8+ lymphocytes at the time of the baseline examination. No significant differences were observed between the placebo and APE groups in these parameters.

Table 2. Demographic and baseline characteristics of full analysis set.

			Placebo N = 55		APE N = 53		
			Mean	**SD**	**Mean**	**SD**	***p* Value**
Sex	Male	subjects	28		25		0.705
	Female	subjects	27		28		
Age		years	50.1	4.8	50	4.9	0.970
Height		cm	164.47	8.27	164.45	6.72	0.987
Body weight		kg	59.65	11.75	57.32	8.24	0.238
BMI		kg/m^2	21.88	2.86	21.14	2.34	0.145
Systolic blood pressure		mmHg	114.5	13.3	112.7	11.1	0.430
Diastolic blood pressure		mmHg	72.1	11.3	70.5	9.9	0.452
Pulse rate		bpm	69.9	8.2	68.4	9.5	0.372
Proportion to Lymphocyte	CD3+ T cells	%	75.14	8.37	77.27	6.95	0.155
	CD4+ T cells	%	46.74	8.54	46.63	9.43	0.946
	CD8+ T cells	%	21.85	8.06	23.46	9.02	0.328

Table 2. *Cont.*

			Placebo		APE		
			N = 55		N = 53		
			Mean	SD	Mean	SD	*p* Value
CD4+/CD8+			2.533	1.241	2.423	1.337	0.659
CD8+ T cells	High SA-βGal	%	84.84	7.66	85.16	8.85	0.840
	Naïve	%	18.47	9.43	17.54	7.65	0.578
	Central memory	%	16.21	10.29	14.07	7.6	0.221
	Effector memory	%	38.89	11.77	39.8	12.18	0.694
	TEMRA	%	26.43	14.9	28.59	13.91	0.439
	PD-1+	%	8.180	6.040	7.680	5.050	0.638
CD4+ T cells	High SA-βGal	%	53.7	17.59	54.83	16.47	0.732
	Naïve	%	24.36	12.71	22.8	10.44	0.489
	Central memory	%	53.57	11.61	52.81	10.95	0.727
	Effector memory	%	21.09	7.77	23.32	10.61	0.218
	TEMRA	%	0.981	2.062	1.071	1.549	0.798
	PD-1+	%	14.360	4.820	14.980	5.580	0.542

Values are represented as means ± SDs. Placebo and APE mean Placebo and APE groups, respectively. Student's *t*-test was used to compare Placebo and APE. Sex was compared using Fisher's exact test.

3.2. Primary and Secondary Outcome Measures

The changes in the values of the primary and secondary endpoints from baseline are shown in Tables 3 and S1 and Figures 2 and 3. The proportion of high-SA-βGal CD8+ T cells decreased after treatment intake in both the placebo and APE groups, with no significant differences between groups (Table 3). As for the secondary endpoints, the proportion of naïve CD4+ T cells tended to increase in the APE group and the proportion of CD3+ T cells in lymphocytes tended to be higher in the placebo group than in the APE group; however, no significant differences were observed (Table S1, Figure 2). For the proportion of PD-1-positive CD8+ T cells, both groups showed approximately 6% higher proportions at eight weeks compared to the baseline. The evaluation of PD-1-positive CD8+ T cell measurements at the 8-week point was put on hold due to the lack of consistency in the data compared to other time points (Table S1).

Table 3. The changes in the proportion of high-SA-βGal-expressing T cells.

					Time After Start of Intake of Trial Supplement					
					Baseline		4 Weeks		8 Weeks	
					Mean	SE	Mean	SE	Mean	SE
Overall	High-SA-βGal CD8+	%	Placebo	N = 55	84.84	1.03	−2.07	1.01	−5.25	1.20
			APE	N = 53	85.16	1.22	−3.02	0.96	−6.92	1.12
			p value		0.840		0.499		0.311	
	High-SA-βGal CD4+	%	Placebo	N = 55	53.70	17.59	−6.37	1.84	−15.82	1.41
			APE	N = 53	54.83	16.47	−7.29	1.70	−16.91	1.67
			p value		0.732		0.715		0.618	
Male	High-SA-βGal CD8+	%	Placebo	N = 28	85.06	1.26	−1.13	1.26	−4.01	1.18
			APE	N = 25	86.08	1.31	−3.00	1.27	−8.20	1.69
			p value		0.575		0.303		0.044	
	High-SA-βGal CD4+	%	Placebo	N = 28	53.09	3.62	−4.82	2.07	−14.19	1.78
			APE	N = 25	55.00	2.94	−7.11	2.15	−16.37	1.88
			p value		0.689		0.447		0.404	

Table 3. *Cont.*

					Time After Start of Intake of Trial Supplement					
					Baseline		4 Weeks		8 Weeks	
					Mean	SE	Mean	SE	Mean	SE
Female	High-SA-βGal CD8+	%	Placebo	N = 27	84.61	1.67	−3.05	1.60	−6.54	2.12
			APE	N = 28	84.34	2.00	−3.04	1.44	−5.78	1.47
			p value		0.918		0.997		0.770	
	High-SA-βGal CD4+	%	Placebo	N = 27	54.34	3.10	−7.97	3.09	−17.50	2.20
			APE	N = 28	54.68	3.44	−7.45	2.62	−17.39	2.71
			p value		0.941		0.897		0.975	

Values are represented as means ± SEs. Placebo and APE mean Placebo and APE groups, respectively. Between-group comparisons were assessed by Student's *t*-tests. The baseline values represent the measured values, while the values at 4 and 8 weeks indicate changes from baseline.

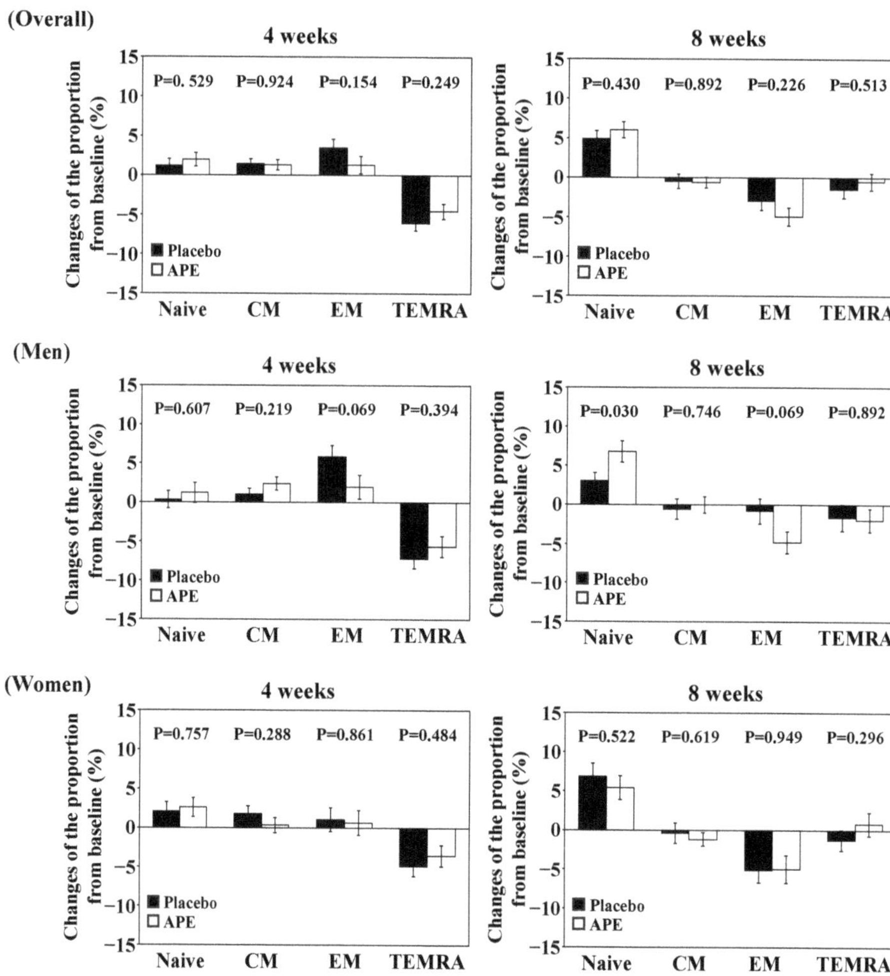

Figure 2. The changes in the proportion of subsets of CD8+ T cells. Values are represented as means ± SDs. Placebo and APE mean Placebo and APE groups, respectively. Note that "4 weeks" and "8 weeks" indicate the time points (in weeks) after the start of trial supplement intake. "Naive", "CM", "EM", and "TEMRA" mean naive T cell, central memory T cell, effector memory T cell, and TEMRA cell, respectively. Student's *t*-test was used to compare Placebo and APE. The *p*-values are shown in the graphs.

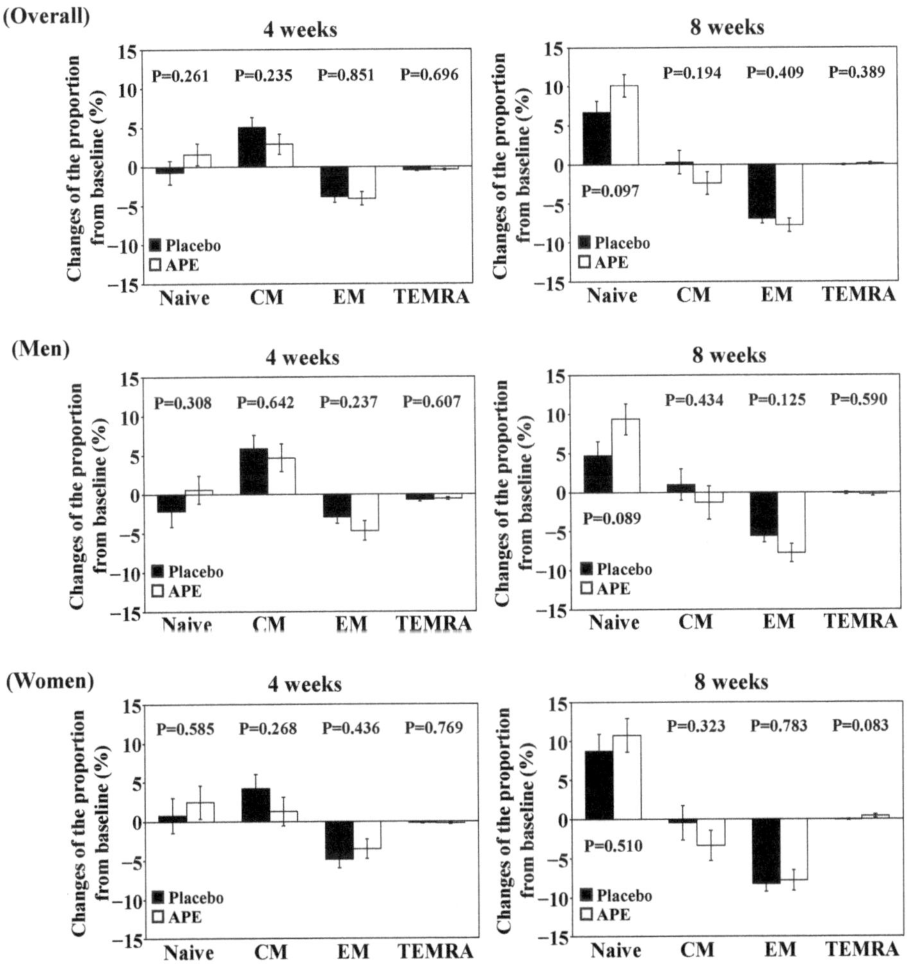

Figure 3. The changes in the proportion of subsets of CD4+ T cells. Values are represented as means ± SDs. Placebo and APE mean Placebo and APE groups, respectively. Note that "4 weeks" and "8 weeks" indicate the time points (in weeks) after the start of trial supplement intake. "Naive", "CM", "EM", and "TEMRA" means naive T cell, central memory T cell, effector memory T cell, and TEMRA cell, respectively. Student's *t*-test was used to compare Placebo and APE. The *p*-values are shown in the graphs.

3.3. Subgroup Analysis

The results of the subgroup analysis according to sex are shown in Tables 3 and S1, Figures 2 and 3. In terms of the proportion of high-SA-βGal CD8+ T cells in male subjects, both groups showed a decrease at 8 weeks from the baseline; however, the APE group showed significantly lower values than the placebo group at the same period (Table 3). In contrast, for females, both groups showed a decrease at 8 weeks from the baseline, but there was no significant difference between the groups (Table 3).

The CD8+ T cell/lymphocyte ratio was significantly lower in males in the placebo group than in the APE group at baseline, resulting in significantly higher baseline values for the CD4+/CD8+ cell ratio in the placebo group than in the APE group (Table S1B). Therefore, an ANCOVA with the baseline value as a covariate was conducted. No differences were observed between the placebo and APE groups in the CD8+ T cell/lymphocyte ratio and the CD4+/CD8+ ratio (p = 0.6546 and 0.1378, respectively). Although a significant difference was observed in the CD4+/CD8+ ratio among females (p = 0.048), the ANCOVA showed no significant difference (p = 0.0875).

For the T cell subset, the proportion of naïve CD8+ T cells in males increased in both groups after the start of intake but became significantly higher in the APE group than in the placebo group at 8 weeks (Table S1, Figure 2). In contrast, the proportion of effector memory CD8+ T cells decreased from baseline to 8 weeks in the APE group, whereas the placebo group showed little change from baseline. At 8 weeks, the APE group showed a lower value than the placebo group (ANCOVA, p = 0.0462). This suggests that the increase in the number of naïve T cells was due to the removal of senescent effector memory CD8+ T cells. No significant differences between the groups were observed in other parameters or in females (Table S1, Figure 2).

3.4. Exploratory Efficacy Analysis

For exploratory efficacy evaluation, the gene expression levels of p16, p21, p53, and Sirt1 in the PBMC population were measured using absolute quantification via dPCR. The results showed no movement linked to changes in high-SA-βGal CD8+ T cells (Table S2).

3.5. Safety

Table 4 lists the adverse events observed in this study. There were 15 adverse events reported in 14 of 55 subjects in the placebo group and 22 adverse events in 14 of the 54 subjects in the APE group.

Table 4. List of adverse events.

		Placebo N = 55	APE N = 54
Proportion of subjects with adverse events	%	25.5	25.9
Total number of adverse events	cases	15 (3)	22 (3)
COVID-19	cases	0	1 (1)
Influenza A (headache)	cases	0	1
Meibomian gland infarction (lower left eyelid)	cases	0	1 (1)
Common cold symptoms (sore throat)	cases	0	1
Cold-like symptoms (fatigue)	cases	0	1 (1)
Cold-like symptoms (fatigue, nasal discharge)	cases	0	1
Common cold symptoms (fatigue, fever)	cases	1	0
Common cold symptoms (sore throat, cough, joint pain)	cases	1	0
Sore throat, nasal discharge	cases	0	1
Nasal discharge	cases	2	1
Nasal discharge, headache	cases	0	1
Cough	cases	1 (1)	0
Cough, hoarseness	cases	0	1
Fever	cases	1	1
Fever, cough	cases	1	0
Gingivitis	cases	1	0
Stomach pain	cases	1	0
Abdominal pain	cases	0	2
Soft stool	cases	1	0
Diarrhea	cases	2	0
Occipital neuralgia	cases	0	1
Headache	cases	2 (2)	3
Headache, vomiting	cases	1	0

Table 4. *Cont.*

		Placebo N = 55	APE N = 54
Migraine	cases	0	1
Dizziness	cases	0	1
Vertigo	cases	0	1
Fatigue	cases	0	1
Joint pain (shoulder, arm)	cases	0	1

Numbers in parentheses indicate adverse events that occurred prior to intake of trial supplements.

All adverse events were mild, and the symptoms were resolved during this study. The principal investigational doctor judged that these adverse events were unrelated to the trial supplements and that no side effects were observed. Additionally, although significant changes were observed in the individual clinical test values and the average clinical test values for each group, the principal investigational doctor judged these changes to be clinically insignificant.

4. Discussion

Geroscience is a concept that revolves around the notion that targeting the aging process can have the greatest impact on human health because aging is the greatest risk factor for many diseases [37]. Cellular senescence, one of the 15 hallmarks of aging, is vital because of its impact on aging through the cessation of cell proliferation, decline in cell function, and secretion of SASP factors [11]. Senolytic agents have been studied as a means of combating cellular senescence. For example, quercetin plus dasatinib, BCL2 inhibitors, BET (bromodomain and extra-terminal domain) inhibitors, and fisetin are expected to act as senolytics [14,38,39]. Although studies have investigated senolytic agents and their anti-aging effects in humans, their number remains limited [40]. *A. pilosa* Ledeb., a traditional medicinal herb, has been confirmed to have senolytic effects in vivo, making it a promising candidate as an oral senolytic food ingredient [32]. However, like other potential senolytic agents, its effects on humans remain unclear. Therefore, we conducted a randomized, double-blind, placebo-controlled, parallel-group comparison study in which middle-aged Japanese subjects with immunosenescence continuously consumed APE for eight weeks.

The efficacy of APE was not observed in the overall population; however, APE intake was suggested to reduce high-SA-βGal CD8+ T cells in the male population. The populations of high-SA-βGal CD8+ T cells were presumed to be memory T cells and TEMRA T cells. Additionally, among memory T cells, effector memory T cells express higher levels of SA-βGal than central memory T cells [23]. In this study, the consumption of APE resulted in little change in the proportion of central memory T cells; however, the proportion of effector memory T cells decreased while that of naïve T cells increased. This suggests that the consumption of APE may eliminate effector memory CD8+ T cells that highly express SA-βGal and are undergoing aging. Martínez-Zamudio et al. reported that the high-SA-βGal CD8+ T cell population showed characteristics of senescence induced by telomere dysfunction and p16-mediated senescence. Based on this, the reduction in high-SA-βGal CD8+ T cells observed with APE intake in this study was presumed to reflect its senolytic effects. However, to more accurately evaluate the senolytic effects of APE, it would be appropriate to assess senescent T cell markers (e.g., KLRG1 (killer cell lectin-like receptor G1)), and SASP factors would be useful for evaluating the senolytic effects of APE [41].

In a previous study, the administration of APE to aged mice was reported to decrease the gene expression levels of p16 and p53 [32]. However, in this study, we observed no impact of APE intake on the expression of these genes and Sirt1. One possible explanation is that APE exerts only a limited effect on senescent cells. Another consideration is that the

PBMC population used here for gene expression analysis was composed not only of CD3+ T cells but also B cells, NK cells, monocytes, and dendritic cells. The presence of these additional cell types, beyond CD8+ T cells, may have obscured any potential APE-induced effects [42].

In this study, a decrease in high-SA-βGal CD8+ T cells, an increase in naïve CD8+ T cells, and a decrease in effector memory CD8+ T cells were observed in males following APE intake, whereas these effects were not observed in females. In women, hormones such as estrogen (specifically, estradiol), progesterone, and their regulatory factors (e.g., follicle-stimulating hormone [FSH] and luteinizing hormone [LH]) have well-documented effects on immune cell function and senescence [43–46]. Estrogen, for instance, not only modulates the expression of senescence-related proteins but also influences the differentiation and activation of T cells [44,45]. Estrogen receptors are also expressed on CD8+ T cells, and it has been reported that estrogen analogs can induce antitumor immunity [47]. Indeed, the fluctuation in serum levels of these hormones between premenopausal, perimenopausal, and postmenopausal women could result in variable responses to senolytic interventions with APE. For instance, Fang et al. reported that when fisetin and dasatinib plus quercetin were administered to male and female mice, respectively, the treatment was effective in reducing SASP in male mice, whereas it had no effect or even a harmful effect in female mice [48]. They speculated that the difference in the effectiveness of these senolytics between males and females may be due to the slower biological aging process in females compared to males [48]. Since sex hormones, particularly estrogen, have been shown to have anti-aging effects, future research should measure sex hormone levels, such as estrogen, and investigate their potential influence on the effects of APE on senescent cells.

The targets of senolytic agents have been proposed to include anti-apoptotic proteins of senescent cells (e.g., the BCL-2 family), organelles such as mitochondria that have become dysfunctional in senescent cells, surface antigens of senescent cells, membrane potentials, and other specific biochemical changes [49,50]. Dasatinib, a tyrosine kinase inhibitor and a specific inhibitor of the anti-apoptotic proteins BCL-2 and BCL-xL, induces apoptosis by suppressing the ERK-AKT signaling pathway, thereby inducing senolysis [51,52]. *A. pilosa* Ledeb. contains over 250 substances, including flavonoids, phenolic compounds, phloroglucinol derivatives, tannins, and pentacyclic triterpenoids [24,25]. It has been reported that APE and its constituent compounds induce apoptosis in cancer cells by activating Bax and caspase-3 and inhibiting the ERK-AKT signaling pathway [53,54]. Dryocrassin ABBA, a phloroglucinol derived from *Dryopteris crassirhizoma*, induces apoptosis in liver cancer cell lines by simultaneously inhibiting BCL-2 expression and increasing Bax expression [55]. Agrimols, a characteristic phloroglucinol contained in APE, also reduce the proportion of SA-βGal-positive doxorubicin-induced senescent WI-38 cells by inducing apoptosis. Therefore, we speculated that agrimols are the active substances responsible for the senolytic effects of APE [32]. The mechanism of APE senolysis is not clear, but APE may exhibit senolysis via a mechanism similar to that of dasatinib and navitoclax (ABT-263).

Mitochondrial function is impaired in senescent cells, so it can be targeted by senolytic treatments. Agrimol B activates the Sirtuin/Nrf2 pathway [56]. Nrf2 activation contributes to mitochondrial biogenesis and energy production, enhancing mitochondrial function [57,58]. Therefore, agrimol B may indirectly enhance mitochondrial function. In contrast, agrimol B has been reported to induce apoptosis in tumor cells by inhibiting mitochondrial function by binding to PGC-1α (peroxisome proliferator-activated receptor gamma coactivator 1-alpha) [59]. Thus, although agrimol B may have opposing effects on mitochondria, it may induce apoptosis in senescent cells by inhibiting mitochondrial function.

Although various studies on senolytic agents have been conducted, few reports have verified their effects in humans [6]. In this context, the results of this study suggesting the senolytic effects of APE intake are expected to serve as preliminary insights for the development of senolytic agents. However, further investigation is needed to clarify the senolytic effects of APE. Moreover, even if the senolytic effects of APE are confirmed, its impact on age-related diseases remains unclear. For example, patients with bipolar disorder show decreased proportions of naïve T cells, increased proportions of memory and senescent T cells, and inflammation throughout the body [60]. Additionally, cytotoxic CD8+ cells can infiltrate the brain and have been implicated in inflammatory and degenerative brain diseases [61]. These reports indicate that the clearance of senescent CD8+ T cells by APE may affect the central nervous system. Indeed, our research group has confirmed that the administration of APE improves mood states such as vigor and fatigue in middle-aged Japanese people experiencing poor mood states [62]. Given these preliminary findings, further investigation into the senolytic effects of APE, particularly in the context of sex-specific hormonal influences, is warranted.

5. Conclusions

In this study, an *A. pilosa* extract containing agrimols (APE) was administered to men and women aged 40 to under 60 years with immunosenescence. Our findings indicated that the intake of APE in the overall population did not significantly reduce senescent immune cells (high-SA-βGal CD8+ T cells). However, a potential reduction in high-SA-βGal CD8+ T cells was observed in men, suggesting a possible sex-dependent effect of APE on immunosenescence. The effect of APE on the expression of cell cycle markers and the *Sirt1* gene was not observed, which was likely due to the heterogeneous cell population used for measurement. These results, while preliminary, underscore the importance of evaluating additional senescence markers, SASP factors, and oxidative stress markers to clarify the mechanism of APE's effects. Moreover, since the degree and mechanism by which APE reduces senescent cells may differ between men and women, further investigation is needed into potential sex differences, including the measurement of sex hormones such as estrogen and progesterone, in future studies.

Furthermore, our finding highlights the need to integrate mechanistic in vitro studies, in vivo animal experiments, and larger-scale human trials to determine whether APE can effectively mitigate immunosenescence and serve as a targeted intervention for age-related immune decline.

6. Limitations

This study has several limitations. First, the effectiveness of APE (containing agrimols) in individuals aged 60 and above remains unclear, as the current investigation focused on those aged 40 to under 60. Second, although a reduction in high-SA-βGal CD8+ T cells was found only in males, the factors contributing to this potential sex-specific response—particularly in females—were not fully explored. Third, we focused on SA-βGal as a senescent marker without assessing other markers such as KLRG1, oxidative stress markers, and SASP factors (e.g., IL-1β, IL-6), making it difficult to obtain a comprehensive picture of APE's effect on the senescence phenotype. Similarly, the effects of APE on cell cycle markers in the CD8+ T cell population could not be investigated, leaving the mechanisms underlying its potential senolytic activity unresolved. Fourth, while this study highlights an impact on cellular senescence within the context of immunosenescence, its relevance to aging-related diseases remains unknown. Thus, additional research is needed to clarify whether APE can modulate aging pathways beyond immunosenescence parameters.

Furthermore, this study did not systematically evaluate the role of sex hormones such as estrogen and progesterone, which may affect the senolytic effects. Accounting for these hormonal influences is critical to fully understanding the observed sex-specific tendency of APE's effects. Future studies should include a more diverse age range, multiple senescence markers and SASP factors, and detailed investigations of mitochondrial function and apoptosis-related molecules (e.g., BCL-2, Bax). Such comprehensive studies will help elucidate the mechanisms underlying APE's potential senolytic effects, determine whether distinct effects exist between males and females, and establish its potential utility in mitigating both immunosenescence and age-related disease. Therefore, further research with improvements in study design and evaluation parameters is necessary to validate and expand upon our preliminary findings.

Supplementary Materials: The following supporting information can be downloaded at: https://www.mdpi.com/article/10.3390/nu17040667/s1, Table S1: The Changes in T lymphocyte proportions and its subsets; Table S2: The gene expression of cell cycle markers and Sirt1 in the PBMC population.

Author Contributions: Conceptualization: Y.S., M.H., T.S., Y.I.; Data curation: Y.S., S.S.; Formal analysis: Y.S., S.S.; Funding acquisition: T.W., Y.I., S.T.; Investigation: Y.S., S.S., M.H., M.Y., T.W., Y.H., J.S.; Methodology: Y.S., M.H., Y.I.; Project administration: T.W., Y.I., S.T.; Resources: Y.H., J.S.; Supervision: S.T.; Visualization: Y.S., S.S.; Writing—original draft preparation: Y.S.; Writing—review and editing: Y.S., S.S., M.H., M.Y., T.S., T.W., Y.I., Y.H., J.S., S.T. All authors discussed the results and commented on the manuscript. All authors have read and agreed to the published version of the manuscript.

Funding: The cost of this study was funded by the FANCL Corporation (FANCL).

Institutional Review Board Statement: This study was conducted according to the spirit of the Declaration of Helsinki (originally adopted in June 1964 and revised in October 2013), Ethical Guidelines for Life Science and Medical Research Involving Human Subjects (Ministry of Education, Culture, Sports, Science and Technology; Ministry of Health, Labor and Welfare; and Ministry of Economy, Trade and Industry Notification No. 1; 23 March 2021 [partially revised on 27 March 2023]), and Guidance on Ethical Guidelines for Life Science and Medical Research Involving Human Subjects (Ministry of Education, Culture, Sports, Science and Technology; Ministry of Health, Labor and Welfare; and Ministry of Economy, Trade and Industry 16 April 2021 [partially revised on 17 April 2023]). All procedures were approved by the Medical Station Clinic Ethics Review Committee on 22 June 2023 (approval no. 230622-1).

Informed Consent Statement: Written informed consent was obtained from all subjects involved in this study.

Data Availability Statement: The data presented in this study are available on request from the corresponding author due to privacy and ethical reasons.

Acknowledgments: We would like to express sincere gratitude to the participants in this study and the staff of EP Mediate Co., Ltd. (Tokyo, Japan).

Conflicts of Interest: Y.S., S.S., M.H., M.Y., T.S., T.W., and Y.I. are employees of FANCL. S.T. is an officer at FANCL. FANCL has applied for a patent for *A. pilosa* Ledeb. extract wherein T.S. and T.W. are the inventors. FANCL funded this study; Y.H. and J.S. did not receive financial support from FANCL.

References

1. World Population Prospects 2022: Summary of Results. Available online: https://www.un.org/development/desa/pd/content/World-Population-Prospects-2022 (accessed on 10 May 2024).
2. Beard, J.R.; Officer, A.; de Carvalho, I.A.; Sadana, R.; Pot, A.M.; Michel, J.P.; Lloyd-Sherlock, P.; Epping-Jordan, J.E.; Peeters, G.; Mahanani, W.R.; et al. The World report on ageing and health: A policy framework for healthy ageing. *Lancet* **2016**, *387*, 2145–2154. [CrossRef] [PubMed]
3. Clegg, A.; Young, J.; Iliffe, S.; Rikkert, M.O.; Rockwood, K. Frailty in elderly people. *Lancet* **2013**, *381*, 752–762. [CrossRef]

4. Fried, L.P.; Tangen, C.M.; Walston, J.; Newman, A.B.; Hirsch, C.; Gottdiener, J.; Seeman, T.; Tracy, R.; Kop, W.J.; Burke, G.; et al. Frailty in older adults: Evidence for a phenotype. *J. Gerontol. Ser. A Biol. Sci. Med. Sci.* **2001**, *56*, M146–M156. [CrossRef] [PubMed]
5. Schmauck-Medina, T.; Molière, A.; Lautrup, S.; Zhang, J.; Chlopicki, S.; Madsen, H.B.; Cao, S.; Soendenbroe, C.; Mansell, E.; Vestergaard, M.B.; et al. New hallmarks of ageing: A 2022 Copenhagen ageing meeting summary. *Aging* **2022**, *14*, 6829–6839. [CrossRef] [PubMed]
6. López-Otín, C.; Blasco, M.A.; Partridge, L.; Serrano, M.; Kroemer, G. Hallmarks of aging: An expanding universe. *Cell* **2023**, *186*, 243–278. [CrossRef]
7. van Deursen, J.M. The role of senescent cells in ageing. *Nature* **2014**, *509*, 439–446. [CrossRef] [PubMed]
8. Gorgoulis, V.; Adams, P.D.; Alimonti, A.; Bennett, D.C.; Bischof, O.; Bishop, C.; Campisi, J.; Collado, M.; Evangelou, K.; Ferbeyre, G.; et al. Cellular Senescence: Defining a Path Forward. *Cell* **2019**, *179*, 813–827. [CrossRef]
9. Guo, J.; Huang, X.; Dou, L.; Yan, M.; Shen, T.; Tang, W.; Li, J. Aging and aging-related diseases: From molecular mechanisms to interventions and treatments. *Signal Transduct. Target. Ther.* **2022**, *7*, 391. [CrossRef] [PubMed]
10. Yoon, J.H.; Han, H.J. Senotherapeutics: Different approaches of discovery and development. *Mol. Cells* **2024**, *47*, 100002. [CrossRef]
11. Borghesan, M.; Hoogaars, W.M.H.; Varela-Eirin, M.; Talma, N.; Demaria, M. A Senescence-Centric View of Aging: Implications for Longevity and Disease. *Trends Cell Biol.* **2020**, *30*, 777–791. [CrossRef] [PubMed]
12. Baker, D.J.; Childs, B.G.; Durik, M.; Wijers, M.E.; Sieben, C.J.; Zhong, J.; Saltness, R.A.; Jeganathan, K.B.; Verzosa, G.C.; Pezeshki, A.; et al. Naturally occurring p16(Ink4a)-positive cells shorten healthy lifespan. *Nature* **2016**, *530*, 184–189. [CrossRef] [PubMed]
13. Baker, D.J.; Wijshake, T.; Tchkonia, T.; LeBrasseur, N.K.; Childs, B.G.; van de Sluis, B.; Kirkland, J.L.; van Deursen, J.M. Clearance of p16Ink4a-positive senescent cells delays ageing-associated disorders. *Nature* **2011**, *479*, 232–236. [CrossRef] [PubMed]
14. Xu, M.; Pirtskhalava, T.; Farr, J.N.; Weigand, B.M.; Palmer, A.K.; Weivoda, M.M.; Inman, C.L.; Ogrodnik, M.B.; Hachfeld, C.M.; Fraser, D.G.; et al. Senolytics improve physical function and increase lifespan in old age. *Nat. Med.* **2018**, *24*, 1246–1256. [CrossRef] [PubMed]
15. Aiello, A.; Farzaneh, F.; Candore, G.; Caruso, C.; Davinelli, S.; Gambino, C.M.; Ligotti, M.E.; Zareian, N.; Accardi, G. Immunosenescence and Its Hallmarks: How to Oppose Aging Strategically? A Review of Potential Options for Therapeutic Intervention. *Front. Immunol.* **2019**, *10*, 2247. [CrossRef] [PubMed]
16. Grifoni, A.; Alonzi, T.; Alter, G.; Noonan, D.M.; Landay, A.L.; Albini, A.; Goletti, D. Impact of aging on immunity in the context of COVID-19, HIV, and tuberculosis. *Front. Immunol.* **2023**, *14*, 1146704. [CrossRef] [PubMed]
17. Liu, Z.; Liang, Q.; Ren, Y.; Guo, C.; Ge, X.; Wang, L.; Cheng, Q.; Luo, P.; Zhang, Y.; Han, X. Immunosenescence: Molecular mechanisms and diseases. *Signal Transduct. Target. Ther.* **2023**, *8*, 200. [CrossRef] [PubMed]
18. Desdín-Micó, G.; Soto-Heredero, G.; Aranda, J.F.; Oller, J.; Carrasco, E.; Gabandé-Rodríguez, E.; Blanco, E.M.; Alfranca, A.; Cussó, L.; Desco, M.; et al. T cells with dysfunctional mitochondria induce multimorbidity and premature senescence. *Science* **2020**, *368*, 1371–1376. [CrossRef]
19. Ovadya, Y.; Landsberger, T.; Leins, H.; Vadai, E.; Gal, H.; Biran, A.; Yosef, R.; Sagiv, A.; Agrawal, A.; Shapira, A.; et al. Impaired immune surveillance accelerates accumulation of senescent cells and aging. *Nat. Commun.* **2018**, *9*, 5435. [CrossRef]
20. Kurz, D.J.; Decary, S.; Hong, Y.; Erusalimsky, J.D. Senescence-associated (beta)-galactosidase reflects an increase in lysosomal mass during replicative ageing of human endothelial cells. *J. Cell Sci.* **2000**, *113 Pt 20*, 3613–3622. [CrossRef] [PubMed]
21. Chen, H.; Li, Y.; Tollefsbol, T.O. Cell senescence culturing methods. *Methods Mol. Biol.* **2013**, *1048*, 1–10. [CrossRef] [PubMed]
22. Kang, E.; Kang, C.; Lee, Y.; Lee, S.V. Brief guide to senescence assays using cultured mammalian cells. *Mol. Cells* **2024**, *47*, 100102. [CrossRef] [PubMed]
23. Martínez-Zamudio, R.I.; Dewald, H.K.; Vasilopoulos, T.; Gittens-Williams, L.; Fitzgerald-Bocarsly, P.; Herbig, U. Senescence-associated β-galactosidase reveals the abundance of senescent CD8+ T cells in aging humans. *Aging Cell* **2021**, *20*, e13344. [CrossRef] [PubMed]
24. Qingsheng, S.; Hanchen, Z. Botanical Part. In *Edible and Medicinal Plants of China*; Shanghai Lexicographical Publishing House: Shanghai, China, 2003; pp. 85–86.
25. Jin, T.; Chi, L.; Ma, C. *Agrimonia pilosa*: A Phytochemical and Pharmacological Review. *Evid.-Based Complement. Altern. Med.* **2022**, *2022*, 3742208. [CrossRef]
26. Wen, S.; Zhang, X.; Wu, Y.; Yu, S.; Zhang, W.; Liu, D.; Yang, K.; Sun, J. *Agrimonia pilosa* Ledeb.: A review of its traditional uses, botany, phytochemistry, pharmacology, and toxicology. *Heliyon* **2022**, *8*, e09972. [CrossRef] [PubMed]
27. Kim, C.Y.; Yu, Q.M.; Kong, H.J.; Lee, J.Y.; Yang, K.M.; Seo, J.S. Antioxidant and Anti-Inflammatory Activities of *Agrimonia pilosa* Ledeb. Extract. *Evid.-Based Complement. Altern. Med.* **2020**, *2020*, 8571207. [CrossRef]
28. Kim, J.J.; Jiang, J.; Shim, D.W.; Kwon, S.C.; Kim, T.J.; Ye, S.K.; Kim, M.K.; Shin, Y.K.; Koppula, S.; Kang, T.B.; et al. Anti-inflammatory and anti-allergic effects of *Agrimonia pilosa* Ledeb extract on murine cell lines and OVA-induced airway inflammation. *J. Ethnopharmacol.* **2012**, *140*, 213–221. [CrossRef]

29. Kim, G.; Gan, R.Y.; Zhang, D.; Farha, A.K.; Habimana, O.; Mavumengwana, V.; Li, H.B.; Wang, X.H.; Corke, H. Large-Scal Screening of 239 Traditional Chinese Medicinal Plant Extracts for Their Antibacterial Activities against Multidrug-Resistar Staphylococcus aureus and Cytotoxic Activities. *Pathogens* **2020**, *9*, 185. [CrossRef] [PubMed]
30. Miyamoto, K.; Kishi, N.; Koshiura, R. Antitumor effect of agrimoniin, a tannin of *Agrimonia pilosa* Ledeb., on transplantabl rodent tumors. *Jpn. J. Pharmacol.* **1987**, *43*, 187–195. [CrossRef] [PubMed]
31. Liu, X.; Zhu, L.; Tan, J.; Zhou, X.; Xiao, L.; Yang, X.; Wang, B. Glucosidase inhibitory activity and antioxidant activity of flavonoi compound and triterpenoid compound from *Agrimonia pilosa* Ledeb. *BMC Complement. Altern. Med.* **2014**, *14*, 12. [CrossRef]
32. Watanabe, T.; Yazaki, M.; Yazaki, T.; Furukawa, M.; Izumo, N. Senotherapeutic effect of *Agrimonia pilosa* Ledeb. in targetin senescent cells in naturally aged mice. *Food Biosci.* **2024**, *59*, 103903. [CrossRef]
33. Finamore, A.; Roselli, M.; Donini, L.M.; Brasili, E.; Rami, R.; Carnevali, P.; Mistura, L.; Pinto, A.; Giusti, A.M.; Mengheri, M Supplementation with Bifidobacterium longum Bar33 and Lactobacillus helveticus Bar13 mixture improves immunity in elderl humans (over 75 years) and aged mice. *Nutrition* **2019**, *63–64*, 184–192. [CrossRef]
34. Miyazawa, K.; Kawase, M.; Kubota, A.; Yoda, K.; Harata, G.; Hosoda, M.; He, F. Heat-killed Lactobacillus gasseri can enhanc immunity in the elderly in a double-blind, placebo-controlled clinical study. *Benef. Microbes* **2015**, *6*, 441–449. [CrossRef] [PubMed
35. Dong, H.; Rowland, I.; Thomas, L.V.; Yaqoob, P. Immunomodulatory effects of a probiotic drink containing Lactobacillus case Shirota in healthy older volunteers. *Eur. J. Nutr.* **2013**, *52*, 1853–1863. [CrossRef] [PubMed]
36. Horie, K.; Hossain, M.S.; Kim, Y.; Ishida Akiko, I.; Kon, R.; Yamatsu, A.; Kishima, M.; Nishikimi, T.; Kim, M. Effects of Banafine® a fermented green banana-derived acidic glycoconjugate, on influenza vaccine antibody titer in elderly patients receivin gastrostomy tube feeding. *J. Food Sci.* **2021**, *86*, 1410–1417. [CrossRef] [PubMed]
37. Zhang, L.; Pitcher, L.E.; Prahalad, V.; Niedernhofer, L.J.; Robbins, P.D. Targeting cellular senescence with senotherapeutics Senolytics and senomorphics. *FEBS J.* **2023**, *290*, 1362–1383. [CrossRef] [PubMed]
38. Wakita, M.; Takahashi, A.; Sano, O.; Loo, T.M.; Imai, Y.; Narukawa, M.; Iwata, H.; Matsudaira, T.; Kawamoto, S.; Ohtani, N.; et a A BET family protein degrader provokes senolysis by targeting NHEJ and autophagy in senescent cells. *Nat. Commun.* **202** *11*, 1935. [CrossRef]
39. Zhu, Y.; Doornebal, E.J.; Pirtskhalava, T.; Giorgadze, N.; Wentworth, M.; Fuhrmann-Stroissnigg, H.; Niedernhofer, L.J.; Robbins P.D.; Tchkonia, T.; Kirkland, J.L. New agents that target senescent cells: The flavone, fisetin, and the BCL-X(L) inhibitors, A133185 and A1155463. *Aging* **2017**, *9*, 955–963. [CrossRef]
40. Nambiar, A.; Kellogg, D., III; Justice, J.; Goros, M.; Gelfond, J.; Pascual, R.; Hashmi, S.; Masternak, M.; Prata, L.; LeBrasseu N.; et al. Senolytics dasatinib and quercetin in idiopathic pulmonary fibrosis: Results of a phase I, single-blind, single-cente randomized, placebo-controlled pilot trial on feasibility and tolerability. *EBioMedicine* **2023**, *90*, 104481. [CrossRef]
41. Henson, S.M.; Akbar, A.N. KLRG1--more than a marker for T cell senescence. *Age* **2009**, *31*, 285–291. [CrossRef]
42. Kleiveland, C.R. Chapter 15Peripheral Blood Mononuclear Cells. In *The Impact of Food Bioactives on Health: In Vitro and Ex Viv Models*, 1st ed.; Verhoeckx, K., Cotter, P., López-Expósito, I., Kleiveland, C., Lea, T., Mackie, A., Requena, T., Swiatecka, D. Wichers, H., Eds.; Springer: Cham, Switzerland, 2015; pp. 161–168. [CrossRef]
43. Klein, S.L.; Flanagan, K.L. Sex differences in immune responses. *Nat. Rev. Immunol.* **2016**, *16*, 626–638. [CrossRef] [PubMed]
44. Bouman, A.; Heineman, M.J.; Faas, M.M. Sex hormones and the immune response in humans. *Hum. Reprod. Update* **2005** *11*, 411–423. [CrossRef] [PubMed]
45. Kovats, S. Estrogen receptors regulate innate immune cells and signaling pathways. *Cell. Immunol.* **2015**, *294*, 63–69. [CrossRef [PubMed]
46. Ng, M.; Hazrati, L.N. Evidence of sex differences in cellular senescence. *Neurobiol. Aging* **2022**, *120*, 88–104. [CrossRef]
47. Yuan, B.; Clark, C.A.; Wu, B.; Yang, J.; Drerup, J.M.; Li, T.; Jin, V.X.; Hu, Y.; Curiel, T.J.; Li, R. Estrogen receptor beta signaling in CD8(+) T cells boosts T cell receptor activation and antitumor immunity through a phosphotyrosine switch. *J. Immunother. Cancer* **2021**, *9*, e001932. [CrossRef]
48. Fang, Y.; Medina, D.; Stockwell, R.; McFadden, S.; Quinn, K.; Peck, M.R.; Bartke, A.; Hascup, K.N.; Hascup, E.R. Sexual dimorphic metabolic and cognitive responses of C57BL/6 mice to Fisetin or Dasatinib and quercetin cocktail oral treatment. *Geroscience* **2023** *45*, 2835–2850. [CrossRef] [PubMed]
49. Martin, N.; Popgeorgiev, N.; Ichim, G.; Bernard, D. BCL-2 proteins in senescence: Beyond a simple target for senolysis? *Nat. Rev Mol. Cell Biol.* **2023**, *24*, 517–518. [CrossRef] [PubMed]
50. Tse, C.; Shoemaker, A.R.; Adickes, J.; Anderson, M.G.; Chen, J.; Jin, S.; Johnson, E.F.; Marsh, K.C.; Mitten, M.J.; Nimmer, P.; et al ABT-263: A potent and orally bioavailable Bcl-2 family inhibitor. *Cancer Res.* **2008**, *68*, 3421–3428. [CrossRef]
51. Ryu, W.; Park, C.W.; Kim, J.; Lee, H.; Chung, H. The Bcl-2/Bcl-xL Inhibitor ABT-263 Attenuates Retinal Degeneration by Selectively Inducing Apoptosis in Senescent Retinal Pigment Epithelial Cells. *Mol. Cells* **2023**, *46*, 420–429. [CrossRef] [PubMed]
52. Li, Y.J.; He, Y.F.; Han, X.H.; Hu, B. Dasatinib suppresses invasion and induces apoptosis in nasopharyngeal carcinoma. *Int. J. Clin Exp. Pathol.* **2015**, *8*, 7818–7824.

53. Eom, S.Y.; Kim, M.M. The inhibitory effect of *Agrimonia pilosa* methanolic extract on matrix metalloproteinases in HT1080 cells. *J. Food Biochem.* **2021**, *45*, e13894. [CrossRef]
54. Teng, H.; Huang, Q.; Chen, L. Inhibition of cell proliferation and triggering of apoptosis by agrimonolide through MAP kinase (ERK and p38) pathways in human gastric cancer AGS cells. *Food Funct.* **2016**, *7*, 4605–4613. [CrossRef] [PubMed]
55. Jin, Z.; Wang, W.F.; Huang, J.P.; Wang, H.M.; Ju, H.X.; Chang, Y. Dryocrassin ABBA Induces Apoptosis in Human Hepatocellular Carcinoma HepG2 Cells Through a Caspase-Dependent Mitochondrial Pathway. *Asian Pac. J. Cancer Prev.* **2016**, *17*, 1823–1828. [CrossRef] [PubMed]
56. Tang, J.; Li, L.; Chen, Z.; Liao, C.; Hu, K.; Yang, Y.; Huang, J.; Tang, L.; Zhang, L.; Li, L. Agrimol B alleviates cisplatin-induced acute kidney injury by activating the Sirt1/Nrf2 signaling pathway in mice. *Acta Biochim. Biophys. Sin.* **2024**, *56*, 551–563. [CrossRef]
57. Scarpulla, R.C. Metabolic control of mitochondrial biogenesis through the PGC-1 family regulatory network. *Biochim. Biophys. Acta* **2011**, *1813*, 1269–1278. [CrossRef] [PubMed]
58. Suzuki, T.; Takahashi, J.; Yamamoto, M. Molecular Basis of the KEAP1-NRF2 Signaling Pathway. *Mol. Cells* **2023**, *46*, 133–141. [CrossRef]
59. Xiang, D.; Yang, W.; Fang, Z.; Mao, J.; Yan, Q.; Li, L.; Tan, J.; Yu, C.; Qian, J.; Tang, D.; et al. Agrimol B inhibits colon carcinoma progression by blocking mitochondrial function through the PGC-1α/NRF1/TFAM signaling pathway. *Front. Oncol.* **2022**, *12*, 1055126. [CrossRef] [PubMed]
60. Aggio, V.; Fabbella, L.; Poletti, S.; Lorenzi, C.; Finardi, A.; Colombo, C.; Zanardi, R.; Furlan, R.; Benedetti, F. Circulating cytotoxic immune cell composition, activation status and toxins expression associate with white matter microstructure in bipolar disorder. *Sci. Rep.* **2023**, *13*, 22209. [CrossRef] [PubMed]
61. Meuth, S.G.; Herrmann, A.M.; Simon, O.J.; Siffrin, V.; Melzer, N.; Bittner, S.; Meuth, P.; Langer, H.F.; Hallermann, S.; Boldakowa, N.; et al. Cytotoxic CD8+ T cell-neuron interactions: Perforin-dependent electrical silencing precedes but is not causally linked to neuronal cell death. *J. Neurosci.* **2009**, *29*, 15397–15409. [CrossRef] [PubMed]
62. Tsubokawa, M.; Hayashida, M.; Shimizu, Y.; Sakurada, T.; Ishii, Y.; Teramoto, S.; Nakamura, M. Effects on QOL of dietary supplement containing agrimols derived from *Agrimonia pilosa* Ledeb. on healthy Japanese adults—A randomized, double-blind, placebo-controlled, parallel-group trial. *Jpn. Pharmacol. Ther.* **2024**, *52*, 775–789.

MDPI AG
Grosspeteranlage 5
4052 Basel
Switzerland
Tel.: +41 61 683 77 34

Nutrients Editorial Office
E-mail: nutrients@mdpi.com
www.mdpi.com/journal/nutrients

www.ingramcontent.com/pod-product-compliance
Lightning Source LLC
Chambersburg PA
CBHW062053220926
51850CB00010B/2759
* 9 7 8 3 7 2 5 8 5 3 6 7 0 *